Vagus Nerve

The Definitive Guide to Reduce Anxiety, Inflammation and Trauma with Vagal Stimulation - Includes Practical Exercises to Increase Vagal Tone

Danny Parker

Table of Contents

Introduction

Our body is a wonderful system, yet, many fail to take care of this system well. We let it slow down and become destroyed from within. We mostly react rather than being proactive about our health. Instead, we need to focus on the vagus nerve.

Most of you might are thinking, just what is this vagus nerve? What purpose does it serve? How is it related to taking care of my body?

We are going to look into great detail about the vagus nerve. But for now, know that this nerve is an important nerve that you probably have not heard of before. Some of its functions include regulating blood glucose and blood pressure, releasing testosterone and bile, promoting healthy functions of the kidneys, and even assisting with saliva secretion. And these are just some of its functions.

This book is your guide to becoming more aware of the vagus nerve, finding out how it can help you, and learning the details about it. There is a lot to cover, so let's begin with what the vagus nerve is and dive into its functions.

Within our bodies, we have different nerves. There are nerves that extend from our brain called cranial nerves, and the vagus nerve is one of these 12 nerves. However, it's more than just that. It's not only one of the 12 cranial nerves, but it's also the longest. The name comes from the Latin vagus nervus, meaning "wandering nerve," since it tends to "wander" from our brain stem all through the organs in the chest cavity, abdomen, and neck.

Now, what's in this area? Our heart, lungs, and digestive tract are all parts of our abdominal cavity and chest cavity. The vagus nerve takes care of the vital functions of these different areas of the body.

It has a big responsibility. It isn't just a huge nerve; it's a nerve with a whole lot of responsibility.

The vagus nerve is responsible for your digestive, immune, respiratory, and cardiac systems. However, there's so much more to it. It's vital a long nerve that helps the brain communicate with everything in the body, whether it be breathing, heart rate, or other bodily functions.

There is a lot to this nerve; for the most part, it is responsible for the parasympathetic functions of the nervous system.

But what exactly does that entail? Read on to find out.

Chapter 1:
What is the Vagus Nerve?

Y our whole body, from head to toe, is full of nerves. These are effectively the main reason you control your body and how your body interacts with other items as well: your body interacts with a stimulus, and your nerves report that stimulation back to the brain for processing. Your nerves are also directly responsible for making sure you can control your body; when you want to act on something, your brain processes the request and sends it to the brain via the nerves.

The vagus nerve is just one of those nerves. It begins at the brain and drops down through the body, allowing for the quick transmission of stimuli from the body to the brain and from the brain to the body. We will take quick look at how nerves function and why they are critical. We will address the cranial nerves, thirteen pairs of particularly important nerves. Finally, we will see what happens when the vagus nerve is not functioning.

Nerves

Nerves are highly specialized cells designed to send impulses. These impulses send information from one nerve to the other to get the message to where it needs to go. These impulses called action potentials are effectively the activation of a nerve via chemicals that then sends an electrical impulse down the nerve to pass it along.

These impulses travel from nerve to nerve, much like a student in a classroom passes a message to their neighbor to get the note sent to the right person on the other side of the room. Your brain, however, is passing these notes on an entirely different level. To present you an idea of just how much is going on in your brain at any given time, imagine the following:

You have 100 billion neurons

Each fires up to 200 times per second

Each impulse travels to 1000 other neurons

So, to see just how many impulses occur, you must multiply 100,000,000,000 by 200 by 100, and the answer is 20,000,000,000,000,000. That is an incredibly intimidating number—it is 20 million billion. Your brain is moving around up to 20 million billion impulses of information within a second.

Your nerves are meant to take these impulses from a place nearly instantaneously—and they get quite close. What starts out as an electrical impulse on the end of an axon creates a release of chemicals that interacts with the other nerves in line; and this happens over and over, spreading to upwards of 1000 neurons per firing. This means that the transmission of information flies across the brain incredibly quickly.

The Cranial Nerves

Nerves come in two forms—spinal nerves and the cranial nerves. The only difference is the source of origination. The spinal nerves go from the spine to various parts of the body. The cranial nerves, as you may imagine, go from the brain directly to various portions of your upper body. Primarily, these go to the head, your neck, and torso. Each cranial nerve comes in a pair and serves a different function.

Cranial nerves are usually either responsible for sensing, such as transmitting information about what your body is interacting with, or for motor purposes, or controlling a function. This means that each nerve will have its own primary specialty and will perform differently. When you are reading or learning about cranial nerves, you may see them referred to as Roman numerals from I to XII to denote their locations. I is the closest to the front of the head in origin while XII will be the furthest from the head. Ultimately, the vagus nerve is designated as X.

The Sympathetic and Parasympathetic Nervous Systems

Your body has two primary modes. In the fight or flight mode, your body is incredibly active and ready to fight. There is the rest and digest mode, in which your body is able to slow down and properly process food. These are both a part of the autonomic nervous system—the part of the nervous system primarily ruled by the peripheral nervous system or the part outside of the brain. The autonomic nervous system, in particular, is responsible for the unconscious portion of the body. Effectively, it is those parts not controlled by you but are critical for being kept alive.

Your body's functions are primarily divided into conscious movements and unconscious movements. Your conscious movements are actions you personally choose to do; they are primarily voluntary and not critical to living such as choosing to walk around or actively deciding to go somewhere or jump. They can only happen when you are conscious.

Your unconscious actions, on the other hand, must continue even when you are asleep or unconscious. These are regulated behaviors, such as the heart beating and the body digesting its food. If you had to be conscious to breathe and control your heart, you would literally never be able to sleep without dying.

The sympathetic and parasympathetic nervous systems are a part of this unconscious system. Your parasympathetic nervous system keeps you calm, activating the rest and digest mode. When your vagus nerve is activated, you automatically begin to self-regulate. Your parasympathetic effectively suppresses the sympathetic nervous system, creating a calming effect. It is absolutely critical because your body cannot effectively digest while also actively attempting to flee or fight off a threat. During this stage, as you relax, more blood is diverted to your guts to help regulate and slow down the functions of the body that control healing, resting, and processing food.

The sympathetic nervous system is the one that reacts when you are exposed to a threat. When you feel a threat to yourself, your body immediately activates the sympathetic nervous system in preparation. With the sympathetic nervous system activates, your body is prepared to tackle anything thrown your way. In short, you are ready to fight or run. Blood is cycled through your body quicker as you breathe more, enabling your body to have the oxygen necessary to respond quickly and stay on your feet. Effectively, the sympathetic nervous system prepares your body for vigorous activity.

The Vagus Nerve and Bodily Regulation

The vagus nerve itself is surprisingly diverse. While most of the cranial nerves are designated for either sensory or motor functions, the vagus nerve is responsible for both. It is known as sensorimotor. The vagus nerve receives and sends all sorts of information. Of all of the cranial nerves, the vagus nerve is the longest—it goes from the medulla, a portion of your brainstem, all the way down through your neck and torso, and to your abdomen.

The vagus nerve has four distinct purposes as it brings information back and forth. They are critical in regulating the body. In particular, the vagus nerve is responsible for:

- Sensory input: the vagus nerve transmits feedback from the heart, lungs, throat, and abdomen to the brain to help the brain know how best to regulate

- Taste input: the vagus nerve helps with the sensation of taste

- Motor function: the vagus nerve is responsible for controlling the muscles in the throat needed for both swallowing and speaking

- Regulating the parasympathetic nervous system: the vagus nerve is responsible for regulating digestion, breathing, and heart rate

These four purposes can be broken down into several functions. In total; there are six within the categories of the four functions:

- Triggering anti-inflammatory reactions: the vagus nerve is responsible for telling the body when to stop inflammation by sending out anti-inflammatory messages for the rest of the body.

- Regulation of the sympathetic and parasympathetic nervous systems: these systems are designed to control how alert or relaxed the individual is. They control whether you are in fight or flight mode or if you are in rest-and-digest mode. If your sympathetic nervous system is active, your body is in fight-flight-freeze mode, and when your parasympathetic nervous system is in control, you are calmer and more relaxed.

- Brain-gut communication: the vagus nerve allows for communication from the gut to the brain.

- Regulating circulatory system: our heart rate and blood pressure are directly related to your vagus nerve. The activation of the vagus nerve slows down the heart rate.

- Managing anxiety: when you are anxious, it is usually because the vagus nerve is not able to regulate itself properly, and in response, the individual feels anxious even when they do not need to.

- Allowing for relaxation: because the vagus nerve activates both the sympathetic and parasympathetic nervous systems, it allows for relaxation in certain scenarios. If you need to relax, you activate the parasympathetic nervous system.

The Vagus Nerve and Mind-Body Communication

Because the mind and body are so incredibly intertwined, they need some way to directly communicate. This is the main reason why the vagus nerve is so important: it allows for communication between the mind and the body. The nerve receives signals from the body, and then translates them for the mind to receive. The vagus nerve, in particular, is designed to facilitate that communication. It provides all the feedback for the brain to determine whether the body is functioning properly or if the instructions to the body need to be changed in any way.

Effectively, the nerve acts so that the mind can directly interact with the body and regulate it, allowing always to function properly. This means that the vagus nerve, with its connections to the lungs, the heart, and the digestive tract, is responsible for ensuring that your brain keeps your body alive. Without this nerve, your brain would not know how to regulate itself.

The Vagus Nerve and Emotional Control

Beyond being responsible for your physical bod, the vagus nerve is also critical when it comes to emotional self-regulation. Because the vagus nerve interacts with your sympathetic and parasympathetic nervous systems, it is closely related to whether you are feeling relaxed or anxious. In particular, the stimulation of the vagus nerve seems to have a calming effect on the entire body. When you stimulate the vagus nerve, you are able to directly relax. You are triggering all of the chemicals of the body that slow the heart rate and therefore calm the body.

Think about how people say that yoga is incredibly calming or they rely on techniques such as deep breathing as it helps them feel more stable and in control. This is because it triggers the vagus nerve which in turn triggers the heart to slow down. As such, the body calms down. There is no reason for alarm or feeling anxious. Effectively, the vagus nerve is like a magic switch that enables you to suddenly calm down to get through those difficult emotions that could otherwise become problematic.

Your whole body, from head to toe, is full of nerves.

Chapter 2:
Important Functions of the Vagus Nerve

O ur body functions optimally like a symphony orchestra. Each of the various instruments has specific parts to play, and optimal harmony can only be achieved if each instrument is directed toward doing its job. The orchestra's conductor ensures that no instrument is off-tune or tempo, as a single error could lead to a terrible performance. A conductor that does not keep its goal will also result in a broken performance.

The vagus nerve is the conductor of a symphony orchestra for the human body. It controls the activity of so many different organs and cells, but only when it functions optimally. The body's multiple organs and cells must be capable of detecting and communicating different signals correctly. Dysfunctional signaling can result in a loss of equilibrium in the system, and ultimately a disorder and disease.

The vagus nerve (vagus, from Latin, wanderer) is called that because it is connected to almost all the organs in the body, not just one; it is everywhere. It is responsible for sending sensory information to the central nervous system. It may be considered as the wire conducting electricity from the organs to the brain and vice versa. If that wire breaks somewhere, the organ function will be compromised or lost. For instance, your wounds may not heal fast, you cannot sleep, you eat too much or too little, you feel over-anxious, and the list goes on forever.

Let's break down all of the various functions the human body that orchestra conductor performs for the vagus nerve.

Sensations of the Ear

This branch's function is pure sensation, allowing us to feel pressure, touch, temperature, and moisture on each of the ear's central segments. This is clinically relevant and quite significant, as this is one of the major areas where the VN can be activated, using therapies such as acupuncture.

Allowing Food to be Swallowed

The second function of the VN (the pharyngeal branch) regulates the activation of five pharynx muscles: the three constrictor muscles at the back of the throat and two other muscles that link the throat and the soft palate (the soft tissue at the back of the mouth's roof). These muscles are involved in the pharyngeal process of swallowing, which includes moving chewed food towards the larynx and the esophagus while holding it out of the trachea, thereby keeping the airways free. The active motor part of the gag reflex is also regulated by this VN branch.

Managing Your Airway and Vocal Cords

Are you conscious of the effort required to keep your upper airways open with every breath you take? The muscles involved in this process are also involved in voice development. If you have ever wondered what nerve is responsible for ensuring verbal communication with those around you is feasible, it's the vagus!

The superior and frequent laryngeal nerves are the third and fourth branches of the VN. The muscles above the vocal cords are responsible for the superior laryngeal branch, while the recurring laryngeal branch is responsible for the muscles below the cords.

The superior branch of the laryngeal carries motor information to the larynx muscles to control vocal pitch. The suboptimal feature of the superior branch of the laryngeal results in a pitch transition. A chronically hoarse voice or an easily fatigued, monotonous voice is a sign of poor vagal tone (signaling capacity). Irritation of this nerve can also lead to a cough and the risk of aspiration (i.e., food or drink entering the trachea by impaired vocal cord function).

The recurrent laryngeal branch carries motor information to the muscles below the vocal cords, allowing the vocal cord structures to form sounds by opening, closing and tensioning. It also has a sensory component that relays information from the esophagus, trachea, and internal mucous membranes. Any dysfunction of these nerves during physical activity contributes to heaviness, speech loss and trouble breathing.

Controlling Breathing

What about taking a breath? Okay, the vagus also has a role to play in managing this vital function. The VN's pulmonary branch runs into the pulmonary plexus, connects to the sympathetic nervous system, and innervates both lungs' trachea and bronchi. The vagus component is a sensory nerve that relays information about lung expansion levels to the brain, as well as the levels of oxygen and carbon dioxide.

Vagus tone is expected in the pharynx, larynx, and trachea to open the airway. The pharynx and larynx muscles are innervated by the VN motor components. The suboptimal activity of these neurons can lead to obstruction of the airways, as occurs in chronic obstructive pulmonary disease (COPD) and obstructive sleep apnea. Both symptoms are a sign of low vagal tone and activation of the vagus nerve.

Controlling Heart Rate

Your heart beats to fill oxygen into your tissues and to take toxins away to the organs that dispose of them. The VN plays an important role in ensuring the heart rate stays within a comfortable range when the body is not under threat. Without the VN, the heart would not be working close to its optimum pace.

The sympathetic nervous system activates the heart during fight-or-flight times to increase its pumping rate and the pressure of the contractions in both ventricles. After the stressor passes, the rest-and-digest phase takes over, and the body moves towards the phase of vagal activation. At this time, the VN's parasympathetic fibers slow the heart rate and actively lower the pumping contraction pressure. These fibers work to lower heart activity, allowing the heart to rest and recover from stressful times and severe activation.

Maintaining Optimal Blood Pressure

Blood pressure is an important determinant of the amount of fluid in the bloodstream. The kidneys function to filter the body's fluid and toxins and thus are the major manager of the blood pressure in the body. The vagus nerve relays information from and to the kidneys to help it control the flow of water and urine from within the kidney glomeruli, the kidney's essential filtration unit, while it controls the body's internal blood pressure. When the body is under stress, the vagus and sympathetic nerves draw signals from the blood vessels (in particular the carotid body) and relay them up the brainstem and back down to the kidneys. The kidneys then restrict their blood vessels and increase blood pressure by reducing the amount of water being filtered out through the bloodstream. When the body is calm, carotid body impulses instruct the kidneys to pump out more water to relieve blood pressure.

High blood pressure is a normal condition, and medications are often used to regulate it. It can be a symptom of the overactivation of the stress hormones of the adrenal glands and the stress response of the sympathetic nerves. It is also a very common sign of damaged vagus nerve and poor vagal tone.

Managing Hunger and Satiety

Satiety is attained when the brain receives vagus nerve signals. We require signals from the liver to be satiated, indicating we have enough fat, protein, and carbohydrates in the body. Both carbohydrates and fats are metabolized in the liver.

The following control is mediated by the vagus nerve for carbohydrate metabolism: when blood sugar levels gradually decrease, afferent vagal fibers in the liver increase activity and signal to the brain that more carbohydrates are required by the liver cells. Nevertheless, this mechanism does not signal abrupt changes in blood sugar; these are detected immediately within the brain.

The small intestine releases a hormone called glucagon-like peptide

1 (GLP-1) as a response to increased levels of blood sugar which the body translates as satiety. Diminishing levels of GLP-1 signal the vagus nerve, which in turn manages a slow reduction of blood sugar. Many pharmaceutical companies are now producing medicines that work along the GLP-1 pathway to help manage hunger; however, activating the vagus nerve can manage this within your own body.

The vagus nerve provides yet another road to satiety. After eating a meal, vagal neurons transmit information to the brain about the number of fats, particularly triglycerides and linoleic acid, that have made their way to the liver. This activates the function of the vagus nerve and sends a signal to the brain, which produces a feeling of satiety and a desire to stop eating.

Managing Blood Sugar and Insulin Levels

Insulin resistance and levels of type II diabetes are on the rise at exorbitant rates. Obesity and properly called diabesity—concurrent diabetes and obesity— are big signs of an unhealthy lifestyle. Weight problems and poor blood sugar control are signs that something in your body is working suboptimally.

Our bodies shift their balance towards the sympathetic nervous system during times of stress and release more of the adrenal stress hormones, specifically cortisol. Cortisol's primary effect is to increase blood sugar by stimulating a process called gluconeogenesis when new glucose is created from fat and protein stored in the hepatic system.

Our skeletal muscles require significant energy-forming resources to facilitate the fight-or-flight response—preferably, the fastest-acting and most easily accessible way to form cellular energy that would allow us to survive the threat. Our bodies can generate glucose rapidly and use gluconeogenesis for short-term fuel to transfer it through the bloodstream. The sympathetic nervous system swiftly shifts blood flow to the arms and leg muscles to make us extra strong and fast while shifting it away from the digestive tract and kidneys. We can then easily use our bodies to fight the threat or sprint away as quickly as possible.

For now, it is necessary to understand that nourishment can never move along this path without the vagus nerve. It starts in the pharynx, goes into the esophagus, then through the stomach, into all three parts of the small intestine, and against gravity in the ascending and transverse colon.

Managing the Activity of the Immune System

Would you drive a car with no functioning brakes? A car has the important function of moving you safely from point A to point B, and the important function of your immune system is to keep you safe from attacking your cells and proteins. And just as a car needs a system of checks and balances, like brakes, so your body's immune cells need a similar set of checks and balances.

The immune system can run out of control without its brakes and start attacking human cells, which can then lead to autoimmunity or even stop attacking tumor cells, leading to cancer. A car can be a very hazardous tool without brakes. The immune system can also be quite risky without a system to keep it in check.

Allowing Us to Create Memories

Recent research has shown that gut bacteria are essential for the growth and maturation of both the central nervous system and the enteric nervous system. As described above, the vagus nerve is heavily involved in relaying microbial information from the intestinal bacteria to the brain. This communication chain is responsible for activating the production of a protein called neurotrophic factor (BDNF) derived from the brain. BDNF activation leads to increased neuronal connectivity, and most importantly, to memory production in the brain.

This means that it can be difficult to form new memories and create new neuronal connections without gut bacteria and a healthy functioning vagus nerve. To an even greater degree, if you have an optimally functioning vagus nerve, you are likely to be able to form larger memories and associations with the world around you.

Chapter 3:
Understanding the Vagus Nerve and Optimize your Life

I t sounds trivial, but anything we do impacts our nervous system. The trauma aftermath of the unprecedented firearms abuse and the most disturbing tales of the MeToo campaign have placed discussions of physical and mental well-being to the forefront. More than ever, people are asking what it takes to be healthy and what happens if we are attacked or stressed out.

Dr. Stephen Porges is a seasoned authority on how dire conditions ravage our bodies. He is also a promoter of instruments for restoring homeostasis and returning the nervous system to its optimum degree of harmony. His groundbreaking work began with the Polyvagal Concept, a theory he claimed, "actually offered a new vision of the universe." The way people view the autonomous nervous system has improved. In the last 100 years, our perception of the nervous system has not advanced yet, but Porges' research with the vagus nerve has turned the field on its head. When you have had simple psychology or mind-body relation lesson in the past ten years, you've undoubtedly come across this work and you're already skilled in meditation, relaxation, and yoga.

Why was it so revolutionary? Porges' Polyvagal Theory was the first to foster the recognition and interpretation of the brain mechanisms that are controlled and governed by our bodies. His principle establishes the foundation of the psychology for cognition and behavior research methods.

The vagus is the 10th and longest cranial nerve. It goes from the brain to the lower abdomen and interacts with the skin, lungs, and gastrointestinal tract. The Theories of Polyvagus understand the association between the parasympathetic regulation of certain body processes and sensory experiences of life.

Owing to the unusual connection between our lived practices and our physiological responses, the vagus nerve has become a significant index for physical and mental wellbeing. First, the vagus nerve allows the immune system to function. Inflammation can be minimized, oxytocin improved (read: enhanced desire and connectivity), along with the growth rate of stem cells. This nerve has its effect on almost everything we do. Everything we believe and do impacts the vagus nerve in our body and brain.

Defining the polyvagal principle of the nervous system

In general, the Polyvagal Hypothesis explains the reaction of our nervous system to threats or dangers in three hierarchical systems:

1. A "safe" zone: we feel confident and don't instantly feel challenged. The ventral vagal complex, a brain stem region that controls the heart and the striped muscles of the face and head, reinforces these feelings of health.

2. Fight-or-flight: we feel an activation if stressors occur in our life or atmosphere like traveling onto a plane or experiencing an unwanted noise. The sympathetic nervous system promotes this sense of security.

3. Complete immobilization: what does Dr. Porges liken to the full

shutdown arising from the brainstem nucleus known as the vagus dorsal nucleus. When we completely freeze, suffer extreme or persistent traumatic conditions such as sexual abuse and murder, our biology indicates that we are undergoing such danger to decrease metabolic production. When you feel "numb" or "frozen," like those with PTSD, the driver's seat is our dorsal vagal mechanism, and we behave like a mouse in a cat's jaws.

And what precisely does this explosion of brain and body shifts count as a stressor? Dr. Porges suggests that it may cause autoimmunity and other body disorders such as fibromyalgia, dysautonomia, and irritable bowel syndrome, better known as the "condition of protection nervous system."

Autoimmune Disease and the Nervous System

The sad fact is that we are often out of step with our nervous system. We do dumb stuff like miss meals or scarf down fast food with no concern for nutrition and how everything from memory to our energy level is impacted. Dr. Porges suggests that autoimmunity and other physical disorders — such as fibromyalgia and dysautonomia — may best be classed as "the protective nervous system." By holding our nervous system out of the way of persistent combat, we hopefully have improved safety.

It makes sense that the emergence of "invisible diseases" is correlated with the vagus and the capacity of the body (or lack thereof) to control taxing assaults that are biologically closing us. The strength of Polyvagal's hypothesis is that it provides a structure to understand more how our nervous systems should be controlled and sustained in an environment that advances at the pace of light.

Learning How to Listen to the Body

Dr. Porges showed how our culture tries to accept what our bodies are attempting to teach. Many of us have never been shown how to return to a healthy state when we feel overwhelmed or out of control. Where to begin?

"I'd agree it is a really stressful environment in which we live," Dr. Porges says. "It's not just taxing on social and mental systems; it's always challenging on our bodies. We may fulfil these standards, but we do need time to enable our bodies and minds to be healthy and comfortable. We need recovery periods, and we should start developing resilience with these recovery times. Our nervous system has evolved to perform effectively by going in and out of protection to adapt to demands and recover from demands."

Dr Porges' research influenced his everyday activities and mode of communication. When Dr. Porges grew up, he was a keen athlete and clarinetist — both at the college level. Those experiences became the basis for a revolutionary hypothesis, which allowed him to explore his ability to transcend "dustbowl empiricism" and enkindle his curiosity about the relationship between mind and body.

"The object is everything. Our engine keeps us healthy," he notes. "I did not originally know that remaining relaxed and calming has the potential to reduce negative behaviors. It was obvious to me that kindness and stopping actions would alter state-dependent behavior." Anything can significantly influence our autonomous nervous system, from social actions to internal emotions.

If you feel out of contact with your body and want to function more in tune with the nervous system, Dr. Porges has the following suggestions:

Extend the Duration of Your Exhale

Conscious breathing is the way to start. Use air as an anchor and concentrate on it while you feel anxious or exhausted. Deep exhalation facilitates the supremacy of the parasympathetic organ, which will help to return the body to a stable comfort condition. The enhanced vagal impact slows our pulse, a pace that has a soothing effect as we extend our exhalation. When nervous or experiencing a panic situation, our normal response is to take quick, shallow breaths that raise the heart rate, making you feel less rooted and more excited.

Practices such as meditation and pranayama yoga have vagotropic results that slow down and boost the heart's pumping of blood. The calming reflex by mind-body activities, such as transcendental therapy and praying, are ideal strategies to minimize the release of carbon dioxide and to slow down the body. Continuing the exhale for 2-4 seconds longer than normal would create a difference. Releasing your breath makes your body let go of fear and stress.

Listen to Music and Sing with Other People

A core concept of the Polyvagic Theory is that we are firmly rooted in a relaxed state thanks to the specific (i.e., ventral) vagal pathway, which originates in the brain stem region that controls the striated facial and facial muscles involved in listening, vocalizing and speaking. The mechanism helps humans and other primates to be social, according to Dr. Porges. "Art is modifying many channels through performing and listening." When you jamming to a favorite album, you recognize how easily music and singing can alter your mood. Of note, Tibetan lamas retain elevated rates of carbon dioxide as exhalation is prolonged while singing. Socializing also play a significant part in maintaining the health of our nervous system.

Porges invented the word "neuroception" to explain how our neuronal pathways differentiate circumstances and individuals from healthy to risky without consciousness. Protection neuroception is required before social interaction allows for social bonds. "A perceptual understanding of signals allows our biology to take on an entirely different process that occurs at a point beyond our consciousness."

"We need some social contact," he notes. "We exist in a fragmented, interactive environment, but we crave for social contact in our nervous system." If we are at rest (establishing the ventral vagal path), we are relaxed, responsive to communication, and can adapt.

Bring Awareness to Your Posture and Stand Up

"Standing up affects our alertness and causes blood pressure adjustments," says Dr. Porges. You may wonder why body coordination and stance are stressed during some yoga and meditation courses. "Ground" is a common concept in mind-body activities that implies enabling the diaphragm to be fully exhaled and relaxed. Playing and sitting in front of a computer or riding in a car for lengthy stretches may times to take a closer look at your sitting.

Really Listen to Your Body

You will alter your perception and energy by simply changing your position. You activate the parasympathetic nervous system by preserving proper posture during lengthy exhalation (the way the body relaxes). Although you will think it's too easy just to let gravity do its thing, it takes continuous practice to keep an isometric posture to strengthen your heart and help you relax through any exercise.

Chapter 4:
The Benefits of the Vagus Nerve

The vagus nerve provides nerve pathways to the pharynx (throat),

larynx (voice box), trachea (windpipe), lungs, heart, thoracic, and intestinal tract as well as the transverse part of the colon. The vagus nerve brings sensory data back to the brain from the ear, tongue, pharynx, and larynx.

The vagus nerve as a cranial nerve originates from the medulla oblongata, a part of the brain stem, and extends all the way down from the brain stem to the colon. Total disruption of the vagus nerve induces a characteristic syndrome where the soft palate droops over the side where the damage occurred, along with an impaired the gag reflex.

The voice is hoarse and nasal, and the vocal cord on that side becomes immobile. The outcome is trouble swallowing (dysphagia) and talking (dysphonia). The vagus nerve has vital branches, for instance, recurrent laryngeal nerve stimulation.

Some cranial nerves deliver data to the senses (such as sight or touch) and to the brain (sensory) plus a few control muscles (engine). Peripheral nerves have both sensory and motor functions. In short, the vagus nerve controls many structures and organs, for example, the larynx (voice box), lungs, heart and gastrointestinal tract.

The vagus nerve is one of the 12 pairs of cardiovascular nerves that arise in the brain and is a part of the autonomic nervous system that controls involuntary body functions. The nerve passes through the throat as it travels between the torso and abdomen as well as the lower portion of the brain. It's linked to motor capabilities inside the voice box, diaphragm, heart and stomach and the sensory functions of the tongue and ears. It's linked to both the sensory and motor functions in the uterus and stomach.

As a mode of therapy, Vagus Nerve Stimulation (VNS) sends a regular, gentle stimulation of electric energy into the brain through the vagus nerve via a system that acts much like a pacemaker. There's no physical engagement of the brain in this operation, and patients can't generally feel the stimulation. It's necessary to remember that VNS is a therapy restricted to people with epilepsy or treatment-resistant depression.

People with any of the following might be proper candidates for VNS:

- Requiring other concurrent kinds of brain stimulation

- Heart arrhythmias or other cardiovascular problems

- Dysautonomias (the irregular functioning of the autonomic nervous system)

- autoimmune ailments or ailments (shortness of breath, asthma, etc.)

- Ulcers (gastric, esophageal, etc.)

- Vasovagal syncope (fainting)

- Pre-existing hoarseness

VNS implantation is performed by a neurosurgeon. It takes approximately 45-90 minutes with the individual commonly under anesthesia and done on an inpatient basis. Like most operations, there's a small risk of infection. Other dangers of VNS include pain or inflammation at the incision site, injury to nerves and nerve constriction. The process requires two small incisions. The very first one is left on the top left side of their torso where the pulse generator is implanted. Another incision is made directly across the left side of the neck within a crease of the skin. This is where the lean, flexible wires that link the pulse generator to the vagus nerve are added.

The implant or device is a flat, round piece of metal that measures about an inch and a half (4 centimeters) around and 10-13 mm thick, based on the version used. Newer versions might be marginally smaller. The stimulator includes a battery that could last from 1 to 15 years. After the battery is reduced, the stimulator is substituted using a less invasive procedure that requires opening the chest implants.

The stimulator is commonly triggered two to four months following implantation, although in some situations, it might be triggered in the operating room at the time of implantation. The neurologist uses a stimulator with a tiny handheld PC, programming applications and a programming wand. The potency and length of the electric impulses are all programmed.

The quantity of stimulation varies. However, it is generally initiated at a minimal level and gradually increases to a suitable amount for the person. The system runs constantly and can be programmed to switch on and off for certain amounts of time: for instance, 30 minutes and 5 minutes.

Patients are provided with a handheld magnet to maintain the stimulator at home (triggered by the doctor to a magnet). After the magnet is placed over the heartbeat via a website, additional stimulation is sent irrespective of the treatment program. Holding the magnet over the pulse generator turns off the stimulation, eliminating its ability to restart the stimulation. All of these maneuvers performed with the magnet could be accomplished by the individual, family, caregivers, or friends.

Why the Vagus Nerve is vital

Derived from the Latin term vagus, "to roam," the vagus nerve holds true to its title. From its origins in the cerebellum and brainstem, it winds through the entire body, and branches to innervate all the important organs:

- Pharynx

- Larynx

- Heart

- Esophagus

- Gut

- Small intestine

- Large intestine around the splenic flexure

This long reach results in the nerve playing a part in taste, swallowing, speech, heartbeat, digestion, and excretion. It functions as an irreplaceable member of the autonomic nervous system, or PNS, that is connected with bodily actions categorized as "rest and digest."

As its title suggests, the PNS specializes in calming down the body and digesting foods along with renewing the body's power source, among other purposes. To make this happen, the vagus nerve communicates with its related organs by discharging a neurotransmitter known as acetylcholine that helps alleviate blood pressure regulation, blood sugar equilibrium, heart rate, taste, digestion, breathing, and talking perspiration and kidney function, bile discharge, saliva secretion, and female fertility, and climaxes.

Hormones through the entire body also participate. Insulin reduces glucose release from the liver to invigorate the vagus nerve, whereas the thyroid gland, T3, stimulates the nerve to boost appetite and the creation of ghrelin.

Vagus nerve work is crucial to the launch of oxytocin, testosterone, and vasoactive intestinal peptide. The creation of growth hormone-releasing hormone, GHRH, and also the stimulation of adrenal hormone such as converting vitamin D3 into active vitamin D are given impetus

How the Vagus Nerve Impacts Mental and Physical Health

Even though the vagus impacts organs in the central nervous system, or CNS, made up of the spinal cord and the brain, it's very important to remember that it is suspended at the brainstem and cerebellum. Optimal features, or "large vagal tone indicator," are related to strong social interactions, positive feelings, and improved physical health. People with a reduced vagal tone indicator encounter depression, heart attacks, solitude, negative emotions, and even stroke.

Gut and brain health influence one another, and the vagus nerve is the connection between them. The vagal tone indicator is considered the human body's "gut feeling" which goes straight to the brain and generates a feedback loop of greater positivity or even more negativity.

Emerging studies suggest that the vagal tone indicator is set by signals discharged from the immune system, known as cytokines. Research is underway to understand how stimulating the vagus nerve delivers the capacity for healing inflammatory conditions, such as rheumatoid arthritis, even without pharmaceutical medications.

Advantages and the Truth About the Vagus Nerve

1. The vagus nerve averts inflammation. A certain quantity of inflammation following illness or injury is ordinary. However, an overabundance is connected to many diseases and ailments, from sepsis to the autoimmune disease rheumatoid arthritis. The vagus nerve works a huge system of fibers that act like spies around your organs. If they receive a sign of the incipient inflammation of

cytokines or a chemical called tumor necrosis factor (TNF), they alarms the brain and pull out anti-inflammatory receptors that modulate the body's immune reaction.

2. It makes it possible to make memories. Stimulating the vagus nerves augments memory. This activity distributes the neurotransmitter norepinephrine to the amygdala. Associated studies have been performed in humans, indicating promising treatments for ailments, including Alzheimer's disease. 3. It makes it possible to breathe. Even the neurotransmitter acetylcholine, from the vagus nerve, advises the lungs. It is one reason why Botox - a frequently used cosmetically - may be potentially harmful since it disrupts acetylcholine creation. It's possible, however, to also excite your vagus nerve by performing abdominal breathing or holding your breath for four to eight counts.

4. It is intimately involved with your own heart. The vagus nerve controls the management of the heartbeat via electric impulses to technical muscle tissues - the heart's natural pacemaker - at the right atrium, where acetylcholine release slows down the heartbeat.

By measuring the period between your personal heartbeats on a graph, physicians can decide your heart rate variability or HRV. This information provides clues regarding the durability of your heart and the needed amount of vagus nerve stimulation.

5. It starts your system's comfort response. Whenever your ever-vigilant sympathetic nervous system pops up, the flight or fight responses messages the stress hormone adrenaline and cortisol in your body. That's when the vagus nerve tells the human system to

chill out by releasing acetylcholine. The vagus nerve's tendrils stretch to a lot of organs, behaving like fiber-optic wires sending directions to release proteins and enzymes such as prolactin, vasopressin, and oxytocin, which calm you down. Individuals with a powerful vagus reaction are inclined to recover more rapidly following anxiety, trauma, or disease.

6. It contrasts between your stomach and your brain. Your gut employs the vagus nerve like a walkie-talkie to inform your brain how you are feeling through electrical impulses known as "action potentials." Your gut feelings are extremely real.

7. Too much stimulation is the usual cause of fainting. Should you shake or get queasy at the sight of blood or while obtaining a flu shot, you are not weak. You are experiencing "vagal syncope." Your entire body reacts to pressure, overstimulating the vagus nerve, thus causing the blood pressure and heart rate to fall. During intense syncope, blood circulation is limited to the brain, and you lose consciousness. But the majority of the time, you simply need to lie or sit down for the symptoms to subside.

8. The electrical stimulation of the vagus nerve decreases inflammation and might inhibit it completely. Neurosurgeon Kevin Tracey was that the first to demonstrate that stimulating the vagus nerve can considerably reduce inflammation. Outcomes on rats were successful, and he replicated the experimentation in people with magnificent results. The development of enhancements to stimulate the vagus nerve through digital implants revealed a radical reduction, and sometimes even remission, in rheumatoid arthritis, a condition with no known treatment, often requiring medications.

9. Vagus nerve stimulation has brought in a new area of medicine. Spurred on by the achievement of vagal nerve stimulation to treat swelling and epilepsy, a new area of health study called bioelectronics could be the future of medicine. Using implants that provide electrical impulses to various body components, scientists and physicians hope to take care of many illnesses with fewer drugs and fewer unwanted side effects.

VNS is not a cure for everything. But a lot of men and women who experience VNS undergo a substantial (greater than 50 percent) decrease in the incidence of epileptic seizures, in addition to a decline in seizure severity. This can considerably enhance the standard of life for those who have epilepsy.

Chapter 5:
Vagus Nerve Dysfunction

O ne among all the things that most people don't recognize about the vagus nerve is that it is not easy to tell when it's malfunctioning. Indeed, many people appear to be perfectly healthy on the surface but are actually suffering from a malfunctioning vagus nerve system.

This is mainly because the symptoms are psychological in some cases while physical in others. Given that the vagus nerve plays such a central role in the nervous system, it can be difficult to isolate the pain or symptoms of a disease from the ones indicating a dysfunction.

You're going to learn how to spot whether you're suffering from any of the telltale symptoms and what you can do about it. Keep in mind that it will seem as if these symptoms are related to other injuries or diseases, but the underlying cause of the disease could very well be vagus nerve dysfunction.

Chronic Nausea

I have personal experience with this. Following an accident, there was a period of a few months when I experienced intense nausea, and mealtimes became a chore. Of course, there was nothing physically wrong with my digestive system, and I hadn't contracted an eating disorder.

I just felt like puking after meals or sometimes even when smelling food. Chronic nausea will affect your appetite, as you can imagine, placing your body under further stress. The vagus nerve innervates the stomach, throat, gut, liver, mouth and brain, and it should not be surprising that your entire body will revolt against food or nutrition of any kind following trauma.

Weight Loss

If you're not going to eat thanks to constant feelings of nausea, you cannot expect your body to maintain its regular weight. I happened to lose close to 10 lbs. over three weeks following my discharge from the hospital. At first, I assumed this was merely due to inactivity, but it was connected to the lack of food intake. Being ignorant of the vagus nerve's function, I managed to ingest liquid calories in a bid to shove something down, but the nausea never went away until I began addressing the real problem.

Weight Gain

While weight loss is common, weight gain is eminently possible as well. Some people don't experience nausea but rather intense feelings of stress and anxiety. Eating is a common way for some to deal with such a situation, and the result is a steady increase in weight over time.

While weight loss happens overnight, weight gain of this kind takes time due to a surplus of calories building up. Watch out for any odd cravings you might have or a complete inability to deny yourself sugary foods the moment you get stressed or have to deal with a tough situation.

Irregular Heart Beat

Bradycardia is when your heart begins to beat at a rate lower than normal. Your blood pressure decreases drastically, and you have a problem with staying conscious. Bradycardia doesn't have to be provoked by physical activity of any kind. You could be going about your day doing normal things, and all of a sudden, dizziness and lightheadedness take over. You will also experience a shortness of breath in such moments.

Tachycardia is at the other extreme where your heart will start beating faster than normal. It is a scary experience since you're not going to lose consciousness when this happens, and you will feel as if your heart wants to burst out of your chest. This is what effectively happens during heart attacks, and you should immediately consult a medical professional.

IBS

Irritable bowel syndrome is a condition my wife experienced when she had a bout with vagus nerve malfunction. The reasons for IBS manifesting are not exactly known, but it is clear that vagus nerve malfunction has something to do with it. Constant bloating and an inability to digest food is a hallmark of IBS.

On the surface, it indicates a lack of good gut bacteria needed to break down food properly. However, as long as you're not consuming food that actively destroys these probiotic bacteria, they should replenish themselves (Haas, 2018). Constant IBS indicates a state of stress and dorsal or sympathetic activation.

Depression

As mentioned earlier, gut health and depression are linked (Haas, 2018). Add a general feeling of discomfort and inadequacy to poor gut health, and you're looking at a situation perfect for the formation of depression.

Anxiety

Anxiety goes hand in hand with depression and might make itself known first. You'll always be looking for something bad to happen, and even the smallest issue will reinforce the fact that things are bad for you at this moment.

Chronic Inflammation

The ventral vagus circuit is the one responsible for calming your body down, and it is the one that prioritizes rest and repair. As long as this is being overridden by the other two circuits, you're not going to recover. This is pretty much what was happening with my wife in increasing degrees as she first set aside her own needs to take care of me and fell sick herself.

At first, it was tough for her to understand the link between her feelings of anxiety about the future and her constant pain. Her anxiety only served to activate her dorsal circuit, and as a result, she couldn't help but simply give in to the situation she was facing. Because of this, her body was constantly stressed and never got a chance to heal or relax. Thus, inflammation was always around since nothing was ever being repaired by her body.

Constant Fatigue

Picture this: you're not eating well thanks to nausea and your brain is telling you that everything is going wrong; the best thing to do is simply curl into a ball and accept what comes. You're unlikely to have a lot of energy to do anything but give in to this feeling.

If fatigue has been your constant companion, this is a blaring sign that your vagus nerve is malfunctioning, and you're activating the circuits that do not help your well-being.

Heartburn

This is linked to digestive problems. Combined with the feelings of nausea, this can be a double whammy since not only do you feel the need to puke after eating, but you'll also suffer from heartburn thanks to your food not being digested well. Your body is not prioritizing your digestion enough, and food simply isn't being broken down properly.

The Next Steps to Take

While these symptoms are not serious as one-time occurrences, if you observe one of them occurring for over a week or even a combination of them for the same period of time, make a list and call your doctor immediately. As I mentioned, it helps to seek a professional who has knowledge of polyvagal theory.

Either way, don't delay your consultation for too long since this could cause you to become dehydrated or lose weight at an even more alarming rate. A polyvagal issue or not, you need to prioritize visiting a doctor as soon as possible. Be prepared to reply to the questions about your medical (history) and let your doctor know of any past trauma you've suffered or any history of disease.

In my wife's and my experiences, an initial medical examination ensued. This involved the usual poking and prodding with a stethoscope followed by even more questions. It can be tough for your doctor to pinpoint the exact reasons for your discomfort and get to the main reason for the problem.

If most of your problems are related to digestion, you will likely undergo an endoscopy or an x-ray examination. X-rays are a non-invasive procedure, and it is likely that your doctor will opt for this method first to detect any blockages in your stomach. An endoscopy involves a tube being inserted down your digestive tract with a camera attached to it.

This procedure is as unpleasant as it sounds, but it does give your doctor a good view of what is happening within you. In addition to this, a procedure called an esophageal manometry test might be conducted on you. This measures your stomach's contraction rate and involves a tube being stuck up your nose and left in for 15 minutes.

A more advanced test that is carried out if you repeatedly complain of digestive symptoms is a gastric emptying study. In this, you'll eat a lightly irradiated piece of food which will allow your doctor to track how fast your body digests it. Generally speaking, if the food is still in your stomach after an hour and a half, this points to some form of digestive disorder.

An ultrasound can also be used to detect any blockages in your gut. The test that is conducted as a last resort if your doctor is unable to detect anything is an electrogastrogram. In this test, a couple of electrodes will be placed outside your belly, and your doctor will listen to your stomach for an hour or so.

Vagal Tone

Vagal tone refers to the baseline activity of the vagus nerve, specifically the ventral system (Haas, 2018). Measuring vagal tone is not a straightforward task, but invasive and noninvasive procedures do exist. Often, the easiest way to measure vagal tone is to measure bodily processes that are affected by it.

One of the most commonly measured functions is the heart rate. Generally speaking, in human beings, a base heart rate between 55-100 beats per minute is considered healthy. Any variation from this range is likely to be a cause of concern. More than the resting heart rate, it is the heart rate's variability that is important.

When we breathe in, our heart rates increase and with every breath out; it slows down just a little bit. The difference between the heart rate on exhalation and inhalation is called the heart rate's variability. A lower degree of variability indicates faster vagal response and a higher tone.

A low vagal tone often results in conditions such as chronic inflammation since the vagus nerve is the one that is responsible for switching the body's immune system back on and restoring its healing abilities. In people with low vagal tones, this doesn't happen, and thus inflammation persists.

Vagal tone doesn't just affect your physical functions but emotional ones as well. A research study published in 1994 found that the physiological regulation of emotions was directly affected by vagal tone (Haas, 2018).

The study determined this by measuring the amount of cortisol that was present in the bloodstream of their subjects. As a bit of a background, cortisol is a hormone that is associated with stress and is a by-product of the stress response. Continuously high levels of cortisol in the bloodstream lead to conditions such as IBS.

It isn't cortisol itself that causes this but the malfunctioning vagus nerve that precipitates such a condition. In this particular study, researchers measured emotional regulation in the brain by measuring both cortisol and monitoring brain activity via an EEG test. EEG stands for Electroencephalography and involves electrodes being placed on the subject's scalp.

EEG activity can be correlated to emotional activity within the brain, and researchers can thus match increased activity with baseline data. Prior research has indicated that the expression of emotion and the ability to practice emotional self-regulation is closely associated with vagal tones. In other words, the higher the vagal tone is, the quicker the subject in question is able to return to a healthy state of being (a ventral state).

Chapter 6:
What Happens to Your Digestive Tract When You Don't Take Care of the Vagus Nerve

Our vagus nerve is stimulated both involuntarily and voluntarily. If it's not stimulated properly, many problems can arise because your vagus nerve affects the rest of the body.

It Can Affect Your Appetite

Have you eaten only a tiny amount of food and realized you're full? That's a sign of your vagus nerve at work. It controls all communication up and down the body, taking care of hunger and the signals of being full. When you've eaten enough, the signal for satisfaction goes all the way up to your brain, telling it that you're not hungry anymore after eating a meal.

There are also different neurotransmitters inside our stomach, like serotonin and ghrelin that send feelings of hunger and fullness to the vagus nerve within the brain. As such, your vagus nerve controls all perceptions of hunger, mood and stress levels and the information regarding the inflammatory response in the body. The signals go from the brain toward the gut after you digest food, and the digestive enzymes are all affected.

Your vagus nerve also works on pushing food out of your body, which is another way of saying it controls how much you defecate and whether or not you're suffering from diarrhea or constipation.

This important pathway controls many factors, including your health and weight. So what happens if you don't take care of your vagus nerve?

Fullness Signals

The vagus nerve isn't properly working when you're obese and isn't as sensitive to the neurotransmitters for fullness. This means you end up overeating and not getting enough exercise, causing more weight gain and obesity. However, there are regimens that can change how your vagus nerve reacts to everything.

It takes a huge amount of food to tell your brain that you're full when you're obese. It also doesn't have a very strong fullness signal, so even if you do tell the brain you're full, the vagus nerve isn't working as strongly as it should. If your vagus nerve is stimulated properly, it turns on these fullness signals in both animals and in humans. So, when if turn the signals on, you'll eat a lot less, lose weight, and feel fuller.

Irritable Bowel Syndrome

IBS (Irritable bowel syndrome) happens when you have abdominal pain from the digestive movements, but it can be lessened or cured with the help of your vagus nerve. If your vagus nerve is stimulated, it can help remove waste from your body and reduce pain. Vagal tone controls the motility of your body and helps with gastrointestinal pain, especially that associated with dyspepsia and Irritable Bowel Syndrome.

Insulin Resistance

Insulin resistance is a diabetic condition in which you need more insulin to help break down the body's sugars. For those with diabetes or prediabetes, this can be a problem because it takes much more insulin to reduce blood sugar levels, and they tend to increase.

Your vagus nerve has some authority over your pancreas too, where you secrete insulin to help break down glucose molecules. It dulls the vagus nerve when you're not eating correctly, which affects insulin performance in the body. It takes a whole lot of insulin to break it down, which is why those with diabetes need medication to help reduce this.

Inflammation factors also play their part. When you're not taking care of the vagus nerve and instead are just eating whatever you want, insulin resistance especially happens. When you stimulate the vagus nerve properly, you'll be able to reduce blood glucose and insulin levels.

Gut-Brain Connection

Your vagus nerve directly connects your gut and brain. However, something else is involved stimulating your gut and brain together to counteract hunger and help move everything around. This is called Lactobacillus reuteri, also known as L. reuteri. It's a bacterium that's a part of your microbiome, which helps stimulate food breakdown as you ingest it.

The L. reuteri do this job by giving your brain the signal that, hey, there's food here. This is your gut health working, and it reduces inflammation within the body.

This bacterium helps the neurotransmitters calm your gut and make it, so your body is properly digesting food. It also secretes oxytocin and dopamine, which reduces pain and stimulates blood flow. Dopamine primarily is used in this way.

If the vagus nerve isn't appropriately stimulated, these neurotransmitters won't work, and your body cannot fight off the inflammation coming from your stomach acids, the foods you eat, and the like. This causes a "leaky gut," a permeability of the intestines where the toxins and bacteria tend to "leak" through the intestine walls.

Leaky Gut

Your vagus nerve makes sure that harmful substances are properly broken down through neurotransmitters' function. It also helps the peristalsis of the body. Your digestive tract aids this to protect the body from harmful bacteria and substances. Your intestinal walls are vitally barriers that control the bloodstream and everything brought to the organs. The small gaps in your intestinal wall permit a variety of nutrients to be delivered while also blocking the passage of harmful substances. Intestinal permeability is fundamentally the reason why these substances easily go through the intestinal wall.

When these junctions become loose, it essentially affects how permeable the gut becomes, allowing toxins and bacteria to enter the bloodstream. Your vagus nerve manages this inflammatory response and helps keep everything tight. If the vagus nerve isn't appropriately stimulated, the "leaky" gut happens, and uncontrolled and widespread inflammation occurs within your body, causing autoimmune conditions to take root and fester. For example, bloating, sensitivities, digestive issues, skin problems, and fatigue may occur due to this.

If your vagus nerve is adequately stimulated and working properly, it can reduce the inflammatory response, thus reducing inflammation in the body. We'll go into further detail on inflammation, but understand that your gut isn't just a place where food is digested. It's also a location where a lot happens that isn't fun for anyone.

Taking Care of the Vagus Nerve Through Nutrition

When you find ways of improving your vagus nerve, you are addressing what you're putting into your body. When you have a "cafeteria diet," which involves lots of fats and carbs, it reduces the vagus nerve's sensitivity. However, eating a low-carb diet a bit higher in fat can help. There are ways to stimulate the vagus nerve through a variety of tools, but it's a little more complex than you'd think.

A lousy regimen just makes you feel gross, and part of it is because your vagus nerve isn't being correctly stimulated. A good regimen helps to counteract these problems, maybe even restoring them. We'll highlight what you can do to help properly stimulate the vagus nerve, but being mindful of what you eat is very important. It can help reduce the possibility of leaky gut and also with your microbiome.

It is pertinent to focus on the bacteria within the body. Whether through the foods you eat or through supplements, probiotics are essential for vagus nerve health. The right foods will change the body. You'll have a healthier body with the proper stimulation and the right bacteria and fewer instances of leaky gut or other intestinal issues.

Your brain and gut are connected, as stated, if only through this nerve. Understand that what you put into your body plays a significant role in how your vagal tone improves and how you respond to the world around you. Let's talk about inflammation and how your vagus nerve controls it.

Treatment-resistant Depression

Studies suggested a potential decrease in the symptoms of depression in patients who had the system implanted for seizure control shortly after the FDA approved VNS as a seizure treatment. It is suspected that VNS acts like electroconvulsive therapy by using

electricity to control the output of brain chemicals called

neurotransmitters.

VNS should not be performed in patients with any of the following:

- Acute suicidal thoughts or behavior

- History of psychotic, psychotic, or delusional disorders

- History of fast cycling bipolar disorder

Gastroparesis

Research findings have shown a direct link between gastroparesis and vagus nerve damage. It's a condition that affects the involuntary contraction of the digestive system severely. As mentioned, the vagus nerve, in conjunction with ANS, facilitates the parasympathetic functions of the body. Some of the parasympathetic functions include the involuntary contraction of the digestive system. In simple terms, when you suffer from a damaged vagus nerve, you may never enjoy the parasympathetic actions of defecation. The stomach does not empty properly, and this leads to a continuous pile up of dirt before. Some of the common symptoms of this condition include:

• Nausea or vomiting: This can be much worse and severe. With gastroparesis, the patient is unable to digest most of the food eaten. This leads to nausea and vomiting long hours after eating. In normal vomiting situations, a person just vomits a few minutes after eating. However, in advanced cases of gastroparesis, the afflicted is likely to vomit after several hours of waiting.

• Loss of appetite: Most people who suffer from gastroparesis often eat a little food because they constantly lack an appetite. This condition makes a person feel full even when hungry. Patients However, there are other conditions that may lead to a lack of appetite. If you suspect you are suffering from a lack of appetite, investigate all the possible causes. A doctor can test you for vagus nerve dysfunction.

• Acid reflux: Acid refluxes will occur. However, with gastroparesis, they will be much more severe and recurrent.

• Abdominal pain or bloating: The other direct symptom of gastroparesis is bloating and abdominal pain. The vagus nerve spreads to the lower abdomen, having an influence on your excretory and sexual organs. This means that any damage to the nerve may directly affect your sexual or digestive health. Such conditions will often lead to abdominal pain.

• Unexplained weight loss: There are several reasons why a person suffering from gastroparesis may lose weight. First, such individuals do not eat as much as they should, and the body is denied some of its essential vitamins. Further, the body does not fully digest the food consumed. In most cases, the food leaves through vomiting, often leading to a loss of weight in most patients.

This is a distinctive observation in the severe stage of vagus nerve damage. In the early symptoms, the patient may experience digestive complications, but they are not affecting personal weight. In essence, those who suffer from the early stages of vagus nerve damage still have a choice to make on the types of foods they want to eat. They may still eat without vomiting. However, in the stage where gastroparesis develops, it is almost impossible to manage the effects associated with eating.

Chapter 7:
The Vagus Nerve Reduction of Various Inflammations

I nflammation is the body's defense against injury or invasion. The most familiar form of inflammation is acute inflammation. You've experienced this when you stubbed your toe. It is characterized by five signs: redness, swelling, warmth, pain, and mobility loss if the injury is near a joint. These are all strategies that your immune system is using to protect you. In the proper context, they are all good.

Acute Inflammation

When an injury first occurs, affected cells in the immediate area release chemicals to alert the immune response. Blood rushes to the wound's site, where the capillaries dilate to allow white blood cells through the capillary lining. The infantry unit of white blood cells floods into the offending area. They will search for invaders to destroy before an infection can set in. The redness and swelling are caused by the increase in blood to the area. The heat is caused by the blood also because it quickly came from deeper within your body, where the core temperature is typically warmer than your outer skin.

Mobility loss from the excess blood happens if there's less room for your joints to move. When a decrease in mobility does occur, it makes you less likely to worsen the injury by immobilizing the area, similar to a natural splint. Pain occurs if there are pain receptors in the location of the damage, but it serves a function also. It forces you to protect and treat the area differently, allowing it the time and space to heal. If you don't clean the wound properly, unfriendly microorganisms are given access to your body through the skin's opening. A skirmish between the microorganisms and your white blood cells will follow. This battle may result in pus that collects at the site of the action, evidence of the casualties of war.

If the injury is internal, the body's response is similar but perhaps less noticeable. Blood will still rush to the area. The capillaries will again dilate to release the army of white blood cells for their search and destroy mission. This rush of blood causes swelling and perhaps a loss of mobility, depending upon the degree of swelling, pain, and location. Heat, unless the infection has set in, isn't an issue because internal injuries are already at the core body temperature. And the pain may or may not occur, depending on whether there are any pain receptors in the area of concern.

Chronic Inflammation

Whether the injury or invasion is internal or external, the acute immune response's effects will last anytime between hours to several days, depending on the severity of the issue. On the other hand, chronic inflammation is a similar response, but its signs may be less noticeable. You may experience fatigue, a low-grade fever, random rashes, and dull pain in the chest or abdomen without realizing why.

These effects last much longer, though, and can harm the otherwise healthy surrounding tissue over time. You may even come to a point wherein you are so accustomed to the fatigue, dull pain, and skin irritations that you are barely even aware of them. It becomes your usual mode of operation. This gradual demise is how chronic inflammation can take over your life. Recent studies implicate chronic inflammation as the leading suspect for a wide range of severe diseases.

There are a few causes of chronic inflammation. The most obvious is if it is left untreated. A horrifying yet real example of this was in the news a few years ago when a surgeon accidentally left an instrument in the patient's body before sewing it up. The patient experienced unexplainable pain, random bouts of fever, and debilitating fatigue for years before an X-ray for an unrelated exam discovered the offending forceps. Once the forceps were removed and the lawsuit was underway, the patient had a full recovery.

Another, more frequent, cause of chronic inflammation is an autoimmune disorder. Numerous studies have linked the vagus nerve to this cause of chronic inflammation. Andersson and Tracey in 2012, Tracey in 2016, and Pavlov and Tracey in 2017 have described a response reflex that triggers the vagus nerve to suppress or release signals that call for the immune response army. However, doctors don't thoroughly understand why, sometimes, the inflammatory reflex goes awry. When this happens, "friendly fire" is the result. The body attacks itself, leading to a plethora of conditions known as a chronic disease.

Crohn's disease, rheumatoid arthritis, diabetes, obesity, heart disease, asthma, and even Alzheimer's are just some of the conditions that can be linked to chronic inflammation. During the

2020 coronavirus pandemic, the two most significant risk factors for predicting who would suffer the most or die were age and pre-existing chronic diseases. All of those pre-existing diseases are caused by inflammation. Even age, although certainly not caused by inflammation, is amplified by inflammation.

One's regimen can be a huge factor in controlling inflammation. You should strictly avoid highly processed carbohydrates, unhealthy fats, sugar, and processed meats that can trigger an immune response. People who have spent their lives eating mostly these types of food will most definitely suffer from some inflammatory condition at some point in their lives.

Conversely, olive oil, fatty fish, berries, and green leafy vegetables can all have anti-inflammatory properties. These healthy foods should comprise the majority of your diet. People who eat such items can expect to live in relatively good health well into their old age. Supplements and spices can also help reduce inflammation. Fish oil supplements and curcumin have been associated with a reduction in inflammation, as well as ginger, garlic, and cayenne pepper.

When dietary changes aren't enough to control the inflammation, you can purchase over the counter drugs such as Advil and Aleve that are nonsteroidal anti-inflammatory drugs (NSAIDs). However, using these drugs long term has risks, such as peptic ulcer and kidney disease. If a better diet and NSAIDs don't do the trick, steroids, for which you need a prescription, can reduce inflammation and suppress the immune response. They also have long-term risks associated with them. Vision problems, high blood pressure, and osteoporosis are just a few. There are also instant side effects, such as weight gain, moodiness, and increased body hair.

Another treatment with very few risks or side effects, however, is now being explored. VNS therapy, which was used to treat epilepsy and depression, is now being studied to inhibit the vagus nerve's immune response.

Infection or injury activates the release of cytokines. Cytokines, a type of protein that signal molecules for the inflammatory response, are produced in the spleen. The vagus nerve inhibits the output in a process called the inflammatory reflex. Studies have found that targeting this reflex with a VNS device in patients with rheumatoid arthritis and Crohn's disease reduces cytokine production.

Rheumatoid Arthritis

Unlike osteoarthritis, rheumatoid arthritis is an immune response that attacks the lining of the joints, causing painful swelling, bone erosion, and joint deformity. It begins in the smaller joints such as fingers and spreads to more substantial joints such as elbows and knees. In most cases, inflammation attacks the joints on both sides of the body. In about 40% of cases, tissues other than the joints can become affected, such as the eyes, skin, heart, and lungs. Doctors don't exactly know what triggers this autoimmune disorder. They think a viral or bacterial response may cause the onset. Traditionally, doctors treat this disease with medication, but not all subjects respond to medication.

In a 2019 presentation at the Annual European Congress of Rheumatology, Dr. Mark Genovese, MD, presented the findings of a

SetPoint Medical research study on VNS therapy. The study sought treatments to alleviate the symptoms of rheumatoid arthritis. He cited an earlier study that involved 17 patients with non-responsive rheumatoid arthritis who had the VNS device surgically implanted. After six weeks of daily 60-second stimulation periods, participants noticed that their symptoms significantly disappeared. Then the researchers turned the VNS device off for two weeks, and the patient's symptoms quickly began to return. Then at eight weeks, the device was turned on again, and the symptoms were reduced again.

Dr. Genovese then presented the findings of two more recent studies using a newer VNS device model. The more modern device eliminates the need for a chest incision or connecting wire. Instead, they implant the much smaller charge generator in the same location as the coils around the vagus nerve. The patient must plug in a wireless charging apparatus once a week, and the doctor can control the device settings via a smartphone app.

The first recent study he reported had just three participants. They had the new VNS model implanted and were given stimulation for one minute per day. These individuals also, very quickly, began to see an improvement in symptoms.

The second recent study involved 11 participants. The researchers fractionate the participants into three groups. One group received the new VNS model, and the researchers gave them one minute of stimulation once a day. A second group received the new VNS model, and the researchers gave them one minute of stimulation four times a day. The third group received a sham device. Like the two studies, the first group noticed a quick and significant improvement in their rheumatoid arthritis symptoms. The second group, interestingly enough, saw no improvement at all. One participant's symptoms even began increasing. There was no alternation in the symptoms of the sham group.

Crohn's Disease

Crohn's disease is an illness that causes inflammation in the colon and latter part of the small intestines, with symptoms that include fatigue, abdominal pain, diarrhea, and weight loss. It can be debilitating and painful and may even lead to life-threatening complications. Doctors don't fully understand what causes the disease, but they think that a viral or bacterial response triggers it. Certain stressors and foods can aggravate the symptoms.

There is no cure, but there are medications that may help reduce the symptoms in some people. But like every treatment plan, there are some whose disease is resistant to it. In other people, the side effects outweigh the benefits. More than half of the patients with Crohn's disease will need surgery to remove part of the intestines or colon. This drastic measure isn't necessarily a cure, though. Eventually, the condition may re-establish itself in the remaining parts of the intestines and colon.

A 2016 study by Bonaz et al. involved seven patients with Crohn's disease. The researchers treated them with cervical VNS. Five of the seven responded positively to the treatment, but two actually worsened. All of them reported voice alteration side effects during stimulation and coughing, pain, and labored breathing. Epilepsy and depression patients reported these same side effects.

In the May 2019 edition of Frontiers in Neuroscience, a study titled, Anti-inflammatory Effects of Abdominal Vagus Nerve Stimulation on Experimental Intestinal Inflammation, describes the findings of Payne et al. They induced an inflammatory response in rodents and treated it with VNS. They didn't use cervical VNS, however. The cervical VNS had too many off-target reactions. Besides affecting the pharynx and larynx, heart rate and breathing were also affected. Instead, they wanted to position the VNS closer to the intestines. They devised an apparatus similar to the cervical VNS device, but they implanted it in the rodents' abdomens. After activating it, they found that nothing other than the intestines were affected. They also found that the device was successful in reducing inflammation in the intestines. They propose this to be a safe and effective treatment for Crohn's disease in humans.

Cold Therapy to Stimulate the Vagus Nerve

Ultimately, you do not have to continue to suffer from chronic, widespread inflammation. If triggering the vagus nerve through VNS works to aid inflammation relief, you should also be able to trigger the same results using methods at home that automatically tone and trigger the vagus nerve. Another such method is known as cold therapy.

When you expose your body to something drastically colder than your body, you tend to do several things: you lower the inflammation in the area, you trigger yourself to be sleepier, and you constrict your blood vessels, and in doing so, you will find that the heart rate also slows down as well. Effectively, a quick exposure to sudden cold can actually help activate your vagus nerve, triggering it to give you all its benefits.

Deciding to expose yourself to cold should always be done safely, however. Keep in mind that people can, and do, die from exposure to the cold if it is not managed well. You can get hypothermia if your body drops too low below its base temperature, and for that reason, it is critical to make sure that when engaging in any exposure to the cold, you do so responsibly. Make sure that your exposure is short and that you properly warm yourself up after.

Some choose to dive into icy lakes to trigger their own cold therapy, while others may give themselves ice baths. No matter what you do, make sure to use common sense. Do not decide to go and sleep in a pile of snow without the proper clothing. Perhaps the safest way to do cold therapy is in the comfort of your own home with a splash of cold water.

When you use cold water on your face, you trigger the same reaction. You make sure that your body responds to the sudden drop in temperature without having to expose yourself to a dangerous situation.

All you have to do is use cold water on your face. Let your faucet run as cold as possible. Splash the cold water on your face a few times to trigger your body to respond. If you want to be a bit more extreme, take a cold shower or fill your bathtub with water and ice. Ultimately, the method you choose is up to you, and so long as you chose one you can tolerate and do it regularly, you should see a decrease in inflammation.

As a bonus, if you find that your hands are particularly inflamed, the splashes of cold water with your hands may actually help make your hands feel better as well.

Chapter 8:
The Vagus Nerve and Autoimmune Disease

A utoimmune disease and the vagus nerve are as closely linked as inflammation and the vagus nerve because inflammation and autoimmune issues are intricately related—inflammation is an autoimmune response. A handful of autoimmune issues have already been tackled thus far. You have learned about arthritis and diabetes. However, there are several other autoimmune diseases that people can suffer from.

Immune disorders can go either way: they can result from an overactive immune system or an immune system that is not sufficiently active. Either way, there are issues with the body managing its own illnesses as it defense systems fail one way or the other. The end result is that some part of the body fails to engage in fighting off the illness, infection, or another trigger.

The Immune System

Through the immune system the body defends itself from illness or infection. It consists of several different types of white blood cells. There are phagocytes, which attack the bacteria or virus that have infiltrated the body and lymphocytes, another variety of white blood cells. They document the structure of the virus or bacteria, allowing the body to remember the problematic invader and prevent it from arising in the future. Both phagocytes and lymphocytes come in various forms, with each and every one acting as a specialized soldier for the job. Some are trained to do generic care, while others are more specialized. For example, B lymphocytes lock onto targets that need to be defeated before signaling that the system needs help.

The immune system works in several ways in creates three different forms of immunity. People can have what is known as innate immunity, adaptive immunity, or passive immunity. Each of these functions differently, but the result is the body having a defense against some form of the disease. Depending on which it is, people have a slightly different form of immunity with a slightly different impact.

What is Autoimmune Disease?

Autoimmune diseases are forms of disease that develop when the immune system does not function properly and, instead, becomes overactive. During periods of being overactive and running rampant, the immune system attacks the body instead of anything toxic or dangerous. This then directly damages the body, causing injury, inflammation, and suffering.

The best way to treat autoimmune disease is to find a way to slow down and reduce the immune system, and in doing so, the flare-up of the autoimmune disease should fade away, allowing for relief. Some of these autoimmune diseases will only cause problems in one area of the body, while others will impact everything, creating feelings of discomfort and suffering. Nevertheless, regardless of the harm from the autoimmune issue you are suffering from, it becomes important to ensure that the body is preserved in the best possible condition.

Some of these tendencies for creating autoimmune issues can be directly related to genetics, with studies linking them to the families, while it is believed that diet and exercise can also cause autoimmune disorders. One last topic is the hygiene hypothesis. Due to the fact that children are exposed to far fewer germs now than ever before due to immunizations becoming commonplace and the development of sanitizing cleaners that kill germs, the immune system develops a tendency to overreact. Effectively, because the immune system is not being triggered on the regular, it becomes faulty. Despite this theory, however, it is currently unknown what for sure makes people prone to disorders or why they develop.

Common Autoimmune Issues

There are over eighty autoimmune issues you could suffer from. Some of these are common, while others are practically unknown. Of the 80, 14 are relatively common. These disorders are common enough, for the most part, that if you mention them, people will have heard of them.

These 14 diseases include:

· Celiac Disease: A disease in which the immune system directly attacks the digestive system, leading to gastrointestinal sensitivity and inflammation.

· Sjögren's Syndrome: A disease in which the immune system attacks the glands within the eyes that create tears and lubrication. It is most commonly seen as dry eye and mouth.

· Addison's Disease: A disease in which the adrenal glands are unable to produce hormones at the proper rate, leading bodily malfunction.

· Hashimoto's Thyroiditis: A disease in which the thyroid does not produce enough hormones. It then leads to weight gain, struggling to tolerate the cold, goiter, and hair loss.

· Psoriatic Arthritis: A disease in which the immune system causes the skin to develop too quickly; the excess skin develops patches that become inflamed and scaly. Arthritis sometimes goes along with psoriasis, leading to joint pains and problems.

· Pernicious Anemia: A disease in which the body does not get enough protein and struggles to produce DNA effectively.

· Inflammatory Bowel Disease: A disease commonly referred to as IBD in which the immune system targets the intestinal wall. This can present in several different forms that lead to inflammation of the GI tract, leading to pain and difficulty digesting food properly.

· Autoimmune Vasculitis: A disease in which the immune system impacts the blood vessels in the body, leading to inflammation of the vessels, which then causes the veins and arteries to become more narrow, simultaneously making blood flow more difficult.

· Multiple Sclerosis: A disease in which the immune system targets the brain—particularly the myelin sheath, the part of neurons that coats the axon to bolster transmission of the impulse. As this becomes damaged, the individual's effectiveness at passing along messages becomes decreases.

· Grave's Disease: A disease in which the immune system attacks the thyroid, leading to too many hormones being produced and released into the body. This can lead to high heart rates, struggling to tolerate heat, and unexplained weight loss.

· Myasthenia Gravis: A disease in which the immune system damages the way that the brain communicates with the muscles by impacting the nerves that communicate from the mind to the body, leading to muscle weakening that seems get worse when more action is engaged in.

· Type 1 Diabetes Mellitus: A disease in which the immune system targets cells within the pancreas responsible for insulin production, causing the body to no longer process glucose effectively.

Autoimmune Disease and the Vagus Nerve

Remember, the vagus nerve directly informs the brain when there is inflammation somewhere in the body, so it can then influence just how much inflammation is allowed. However, when the vagus nerve becomes damaged, it is not capable of protecting the body from inflammation. The inflammation runs rampant, creating havoc in the body, all because the vagus nerve malfunctioned in some way.

Stop for a moment and consider all the possible implications and recognize the sheer number of people who are suffering from an autoimmune disease—upwards of 8% of the population are believed to suffer from an autoimmune disorder. Eight people of every 100 you pass are likely suffering from an autoimmune disorder or malfunctioning, and because of that, their bodies are directly attacking themselves.

Stimulation of the vagus nerve, however, has been shown to help fight inflammation, which should also help alleviate some of the autoimmune response. With the inflammation limited, the body is no longer sending cues to tackle parts of the body that did not require an actual intervention from the immune system in the first place.

Effectively, the afferent path - the path from the body to the brain - communicates to the body either a current injury or the need for the inflammation and immune response. It has been found that when the afferent nerve is blocked in some way, but the efferent pathway is free to continue as normal, the body regulates itself.

It allows for the continued communication from the brain to the body while stopping the brain from producing more hormones that encourage inflammation because it is not receiving the impulses telling the brain that inflammation is happening and needs to continue. In blocking the afferent while encouraging the efferent impulses, the body has a chance to regulate itself, and it stops producing the cytokines that will create further the inflammation responsible for the attack of the body by the immune system.

Chapter 9:
Vagus Nerve Stimulation for Epilepsy, Anxiety, and Drug Cravings

Epilepsy

Q uantum brain healing relies on a base of orthomolecular medicine including aminoacids, vitamins, minerals, herbs, botanical extracts, Chinese herbal formulas, and many alternative therapies. There is no answer that will address healing for everyone. It is key to remain open to technology when other options have not met our goals. One option often overlooked after trying nutritional therapy is Vagus Nerve Stimulation. This is a medical device that is surgically implanted. Any major medical center in the US and Europe can implant this device for a patient that qualifies.

Vagus Nerve Stimulation (VNS) involves sending a message to the brain using periodic mild electrical stimulation from the vagus nerve in the neck by a surgically implanted small medical device. There is no brain surgery involved. This stimulation or pulse is sent by a medical device similar to a pacemaker. The vagus nerve is part of the autonomic nervous system and controls involuntary body functions.

VNS may control epilepsy in cases where antiepileptic drugs are ineffective or have intolerable side effects, or neurosurgery is not appropriate for some reason. VNS is effective in stopping seizures in some patients.

The implanted medical device is a flat, round battery, and measures about the size of a silver dollar. The VNS medical device was developed by Cyberonics, Inc. The doctor determines the strength and timing of the pulses administered by the device according to each patient's individual needs. The level of electrical stimulation can be changed without additional surgery with a programming wand connected to a laptop computer.

The side effects of VNS during treatment may include hoarseness, coughing, throat pain, shortness of breath, a short and slight sensation of choking, altered voice sound, ear pain, tooth pain, and a tingling sensation in the neck. Skin irritation or infection could occur at the implantation site. VNS does not negatively impact the brain. This is major surgery and should not be considered lightly.

For those with uncontrollable epileptic seizures, it may be last option. Consider all options before giving up on controlling seizure. This is not neurosurgery and it is safer. We have been mentioning epilepsy or seizure disorder throughout this book because it was the primary disorder targeted by the vagus nerve stimulation. Furthermore, many positive benefits of vagus nerve stimulation were discovered while researchers were studying the effects of it with epilepsy.

Epilepsy is a major central nervous disorder in which brain activity becomes exceedingly abnormal, causing seizures or periods of a very unusual behavior. The nerves and neurons are firing uncontrollably, causing erratic and uncontrollable movements. A person who has epilepsy has their whole world turned upside down due to the severity of the condition and the way it takes over their life. A person will often never know when a seizure will hit, which can prevent them from doing many activities like driving. It will also inhibit their ability to go into certain professions. It is a dangerous and stressful disease to deal with.

During an epileptic episode, the sympathetic nervous system is incomplete overdrive, causing excessive and erratic movements within the nervous system. When a person is having a full-blown epileptic attack or seizure, we won't attempt the many stimulating practices discussed. Much more extreme measures will needed. However, the vagal tone can be strengthened to help avoid or reduce epileptic future attacks. The stronger the vagal tone, the better the parasympathetic response will be at inhibiting the sympathetic response. We mentioned how massaging the carotid sinus has been shown to inhibit seizure activity by stimulating the vagus nerve. If this technique works, then it is a good indication that the other methods will also work.

The overall goal is to continuously improve and strengthen the vagus nerve as much as possible. We will not be able to prevent or cure all illnesses. However, as we maintain our vagal tone, we can help to improve the functionality of the body and at least prevent or reduce many diseases. The point of vagus nerve stimulation is to keep it healthy, active, and strong so it has the ability to enhance parasympathetic activity as much as possible. When we increase our body's ability to utilize the parasympathetic response, we will reduce seizure activity effectively.

Most of the research behind vagus nerve stimulation has been to help prevent epilepsy. This suggests that it is still considered a strong therapy in inhibiting seizure activity.

Dealing with Anxiety Using Your Vagus Nerve

How often do you have to deal with anxiety in your everyday life? If you find yourself worrying too much or getting caught up in non-stopping irrational thoughts or even feeling nausea, chest pain and heart palpitations, then this book is for you.

You are about to learn a simple yet very effective technique to deal with anxiety naturally by stimulating your vagus nerve. This powerful technique can be used to relieve stress and anxiety anywhere and anytime: at home, when commuting and, of course, during those horrible work meetings.

Did you know that the FDA has approved a surgically-implanted device that is successful at treating depression by periodically stimulating the vagus nerve? But hopefully you won't need surgery. You can enjoy the benefits of vagus nerve stimulation by adopting some simple breathing techniques.

<u>Singing and diaphragmatic breathing techniques</u> strengthen this living nervous system, paying great dividends, and the best tool to achieve that is by training your breath.

<u>Breathe with your diaphragm</u>: Now it's time to put this concept into practice. The first thing you need to do is breathe using your diaphragm (abdominal breathing). This is the foundation of proper breathing and anxiety relief.

The diaphragm is your primary breathing muscle. It is belled shaped and when you inhale it patterns out (or should flatten out), acting as piston and creating vacuum in your thoracic cavity so your lungs can expand and air gets in.

On the other side it creates pressure, pushing the viscera down and out, expanding the belly. That's why good breathing practice is described as abdominal breathing or belly breathing. Nervousness can be a genuine doozy; it's outlandishly muddled, profoundly close to home, and ridiculously difficult to foresee. There are times when we think our uneasiness is behind us, that we are at long last one stage ahead, then something happens, and we are on our heels once more, battling to return to a position of harmony and quiet. We are the understudies of our uneasiness, and seeing precisely how our sensory system functions and what we can do to quiet it can be staggeringly enabling.

In any case, what does "quietening your sensory system" truly mean? Numerous individuals depict it as easing back the pulse, developing the breath, and loosening up various muscles; however, what really associates these sensations in the mind? You need to know more about the vagus nerve, the piece of the body that appears to clarify how our psyches control our bodies, how our bodies impact our brains and may give us the instruments we have to quieten them both.

Posttraumatic stress issues (PTSD) are encountered by numerous individuals. Ongoing catastrophic events, mass shootings, psychological oppressor assaults, and urban communities under attack add to the worldwide weight of PTSD, which as indicated by a recent report, influences 4–6% of the worldwide populace, despite the fact that most injuries are identified with mishaps and sexual or physical savagery. Shockingly, there is no known fix, and flow medicines are not powerful for all patients.

A PTSD psychopharmacology working group, as of late, distributed their accord proclamation calling for a quick activity to address the emergency in PTSD treatment, referring to three significant concerns. To start, just two medications (sertraline and paroxetine) are endorsed by the US FDA for the treatment of PTSD. These meds decrease the side effect's seriousness; however, they may not create a total reduction of the side effects.

The subsequent concern is identified with polypharmacy. PTSD patients are recommended prescriptions to address every one of their numerous extraordinary and assorted side effects, including nervousness, trouble dozing, sexual brokenness, wretchedness and interminable torment, while lacking exact examinations of medication communications. The high comorbidity among PTSD and fixation creates further difficulties for pharmacotherapies. The third significant concern is the absence of headway in the treatment of PTSD; no new prescriptions have been endorsed since 2001.

Drug Cravings

Addiction to any substance can make the life of an individual go topsy-turvy. From spending a fortune to deceiving one's own family, a person addicted to illegal substances will go to any extent. But how does addiction force someone to put a stake in something and then lose it all? There are several factors at play when it comes to dealing with the growing problem of addiction.

Cravings are a serious issue that torment numerous people fighting drug addiction, especially when they try to come off the addictive substance. Ironically, many people would have successfully attained long-term sobriety if cravings did not crop up with addiction. Apart from being considered as the major obstacles in recovery, cravings are also the root cause of relapse.

A complete recovery from addiction happens only when a person is free from cravings. Living a drug-free life without the need for constant monitoring against drug cravings can be difficult for a recovering individual, but a recent study published in the journal, Learning and Memory, has suggested that drug cravings can be effectively treated with vagus nerve stimulation (VNS). Under this therapy, patients are taught new behaviors that replace their old addictive behavior of seeking drugs.

Role of VNS in addiction recovery

In the University of Texas at Dallas study, the researchers revealed that the VNS therapy helped patients recover from the maladaptive behavior of drug taking. VNS is basically a surgical process wherein a device is implanted to a wire threaded along the vagus nerve, which travels up from the neck to the brain and connects with the area responsible for regulating mood. As small as a silver dollar, the device works like a pacemaker. It primarily works by sending a slight electric pulses through the vagus nerve, which further reaches the brain, thereby controlling cravings and urges.

The methodology is approved by the U.S. Food and Drug Administration (FDA) and is considered as a potential treatment for treatment-resistant depression, post-traumatic stress disorder (PTSD) and paralysis. The study further highlighted that VNS facilitates the "extinction learning" of drug seeking behaviors by reducing cravings and replacing the behavior associated with addiction with new ones. "Extinction of fearful memories and extinction of drugseeking memories relies on the same substrate in the brain. In our experiments, VNS facilitates both the extinction learning and reduces the relapse response as well," said Dr. Sven Kroener of the University of Texas at Dallas.

A drug-free life is possible

Though addictive substances succeed in temporarily alleviating the emotional and physical pains of drug abusers, they have to eventually cope with the painful symptoms of substance abuse. Besides developing a number of physical and mental problems, many of these individuals also become self-destructive and suicidal.

Addiction to any substance can be life threatening. Only a comprehensive treatment program involving detoxification, medications, psychotherapies and other experiential therapies like yoga, meditation etc. can help an individual get sober. Moreover, a holistic recovery management plan is equally important to sustain the period of sobriety and manage cravings.

However, the extent to which health care practitioners can garner results in the treatment for drug addiction is dependent on the clinical characteristics of the patients that vary according to the type of drug abused as well as its quantity, duration, and the method of use (oral or intravenous).

Chapter 10:
Vagus Nerve Stimulation for Trauma, Chronic Fatigue, Obesity, and Fibromyalgia

Trauma

T he body experiences other distressing signs of post-traumatic stress: tightness in the abdomen, a sinking sensation in the stomach, a familiar pain in the mouth, or a constant sense of fatigue. We now understand that as a part of the recovery process, we have to turn to the body. Thus, we have seen an increase in the use of meditation, mindfulness, tai chi, qigong, Feld ink circle, massage, craniosacral therapy, dietary therapy, and acupuncture for post-traumatic stress disorder.

Such mind-body treatments are helping us to be less passive, less aggressive, and less impulsive to stress. We're understanding the options we need to make us stay grounded and relaxed. We feel increasingly more in need of this. One way that mental-body treatments operate is by activating the vagus nerve. Awareness of how this nerve works offers a profound understanding of traumatic stress and promotes our healing capacity. The vagus nerve has, therefore, taken center stage in the treatment of trauma.

Moreover, mental-body treatments are successful as they require structural improvements in the autonomic nervous system as determined by the increase in vagus nerve activity. The vagus nerve reaches through the muscles of the nose, inner ear, chest, back, lungs, stomach, and intestines from the brainstem down. Mind-body treatments change how we relate to our surroundings by allowing us to try new breathing or activity patterns that communicate specifically with other parts of the body. Researchers also calculate the changes that exist in the vagus nerve, often referred to as the respiratory sinus arrhythmia by heart rate variability (HRV). HRV refers to the rhythmic heart rate oscillations that arise with the breath. It's a function of the intervals between beats in the heart. A higher variability in heart rate is associated with a better ability to withstand or rebound from stress.

Chronic Fatigue

If you find you are suffering from chronic fatigue, your vagus nerve may be the suspect, and that is good news. You can activate your vagus nerve regularly in hopes of getting out of this negative loop where you are too fatigued to get this nerve functioning properly, which then leads you to struggle further. Essentially, you need to figure out how to get yourself back into the proper parasympathetic state, and the fatigue will begin to go away on its own.

However, sometimes, the reason why you feel fatigued in general is that you are either finding yourself in constant sympathetic activation, even if only mildly, or you find you are teetering on the verge of a parasympathetic shutdown. Either of these situations could directly lead you to feel fatigued and unable to cope.

It's long been known that chronic fatigue syndrome can be triggered by viral infections, and that a non-stop immune response may result in devitalizing fatigue. For many years, experts in the medical field believed that it is a person's individual susceptibility that gives birth to the ecology for a particular disease state to take form. Regardless, many have thought that the vagus nerve plays a role in chronic fatigue syndrome, as well as a number of other common health problems. The scientist, Michael B. VanElzakker, in particular, argued that chronic fatigue syndrome is a result of the infection of the vagus nerve.

Every time an immune cell detects an infection, it releases cytokines that promote inflammation. These substances are detected by the vagus nerve receptors, which in turn signals the brain to activate fatigue, along with myalgia, fever, cold, flu, bacterial infection, and depression. According to VanElzakker, symptoms of chronic fatigue are the same as those of normal sickness, except they are triggered whenever a bacterium or virus infects the vagal ganglia. The cells activated by the intrusion can attack the vagus nerve by releasing cytokines and other substances that initiate sickness symptoms. This theory shows that the primary cause of chronic fatigue syndrome is the infection of the vagus nerve.

Obesity

The brain may relate how hungry or full you are, but at the end of the day, the vagus nerve is the part of the body that tells the stomach what the brain says. The brain functions as a sort of processor for the body, but if the vagus nerve is sending the wrong signals down to your stomach, you may find that you feel hungrier. You may find that the messages of having enough in your stomach never make it up to the brain or they are skewed in some way.

Because the vagus nerve makes up the gut-brain axis through which the stomach and the brain communicate, it can directly be implicated when something goes wrong. Whether something is failing to activate properly, or it realizes that your body needs more blood sugar, the vagus nerve may very well be at fault.

When it comes to obesity, it is often due to some sort of dysfunctional relationship with food. There are always circumstances in which a hormone leads to weight gain, but for the vast majority of people, that is not the case. Actually, when there is overeating and not enough exercise occurring, it can be a problem. As the years go on, the population becomes increasingly obese. This may be due to the fact that we do not have to be as active anymore. We do not have to run around to make sure we meet all of our needs because we don't have to hunt.

You do not have to make sure that you are able to fight off animals or are capable of defending your family to the same degree that you once did; and because of that, you may find that at the end of the day, you are growing complacent. You are busy with work, so you do not exercise. You are too busy, so you grab a pizza on the way home. You drive everywhere because it is easier. Suddenly, your caloric needs are actually much lower than they would be for a human out in the wild, having to hunt, grow food, and defend his or her home from that hungry bear desperate to get in.

Some people, after gaining weight, find that they just cannot lose it no matter how hard they try. These people may end up seeking weight loss surgery, which is invasive and entirely irreversible. When it is done, there is no turning back. However, studies have found that you can actually use the vagus nerve to aid in weight loss. In blocking the vagus nerve, the individual is much more likely to feel full for longer. This means the individual will not be overeating if the vagus nerve gets the wrong message.

In a clinical trial involving 233 people with BMIs of 35 or over, those who had the experimental generator activated lost roughly 8.5% more body weight over a year than their peers who did not get the shocks. Roughly half of the patients in this experimental group found that they lost up to 20% of their excess weight, while another 38% lost 25% of that excess weight. On the other hand, the patients who did not get the shocks during this time found that only 32.5% lost 20% of their weight, and only 23.4% lost 25%.

These results reveal that there is some degree of promise in using the vagus nerve to curb appetite to alleviate obesity without having to remove a portion of the stomach.

Fibromyalgia

There is still not much known about fibromyalgia, as the pain does not come from a specific cause or area in the body. Many researchers believe that with fibromyalgia, painful sensations are amplified due to the way the brain processes pain. A real reason is not fully known regarding this issue.

Sometimes the pain is triggered by a particular event, like an accident or surgery. Other times, there is no single experience, but the pain just seems to accumulate over time. There is no cure for fibromyalgia at this moment. However, there are interventions, both medical and nonmedical, that can help with subsiding the symptoms that come with it. Once again, our friend, the vagus nerve, is at play.

In a 2011, in an NIH study, the leading researchers suggested that vagus nerve stimulation may be a useful adjunct treatment for fibromyalgia patients. Further research is definitely needed, though. Many researchers feel that vagus nerve stimulation is effective in treating pain because it is able to negate a wide variety of factors that contribute to pain, like inflammation and the pain response.

There is still much that is up in the air about fibromyalgia. However, the results of such studies continue to suggest that the pain associated with it is significantly reduced with vagus nerve stimulation. Pain is often heightened when the body is stress. Since the vagus nerve can lower a person's stress through the sympathetic response, it is reasonable to believe that it can reduce or even eliminate pain associated with fibromyalgia.

Chapter 11:
Vagus Nerve Stimulation for Depression

Depression and anxiety are intricately linked. You probably don't need to know in great detail about depression since you're probably experiencing it. However, it is worthwhile to take the time to understand the biological underpinnings of it. This will make evaluating treatment options a lot easier. In addition to this, you'll also learn how the vagus nerve affects depression and can be used to improve your state of mind.

Your Brain on Depression

Just like the way anxiety is a perfectly normal and natural response in short doses, feelings of sadness and disappointment are similar. Sadness is simply the other side of the coin from happiness, and it is impossible to have one without the other. The issue arises when this balance is eroded, and a person begins to feel only one emotion predominantly.

As weird as it sounds, chronic and excessive happiness are harmful. We just don't see any cases of it because of our brain's inbuilt negativity bias. What we instead see pre-dominantly is a chronic state of excessive sadness, and this is what depression really is.

Depression was never really seen as a legitimate health concern for long periods of time. These days, the conversation around it is changing, thankfully, but there are still are significant roadblocks. Seeking therapy, for example, is still considered shameful in some cultures and men in particular face ridicule more often than not if they report themselves as being depressed in some parts of the world (Koskie, 2018).

As a result, the data on depression is a bit skewed. In the United States, women are thought to be more likely to suffer depressive episodes. However, we don't know if this is simply because more women are willing to report depressive episodes than men. One can understand why men wouldn't want to concede any symptoms of perceived weakness since this is how we're brought up.

It is an experience I've undergone and struggled with massively. Following an accident, I intellectually understood that all the thoughts in my head were false and there were massive biological forces at work. I was the one in control, and I was the one causing these depressive episodes.

However, one cannot apply reasons when emotion strikes. The tidal wave of sadness and hopelessness that hit me left me devastated, despite all the scientific research and facts I had in my possession. CBT, as a therapeutic technique, helped immensely with this since it attacked the problem's biological root by focusing on building neural network forming habits.

Before we go into treatment options, though, let's take some time to take a look at the different types of depression. It is extremely relevant at this point because there are significant repercussions of untreated depression. Understand that in more serious cases, you should always seek professional help. Self-help techniques only go so far when it comes to depression, and this is why it is a bigger problem than anxiety. I'm not diminishing anxiety by any means but only trying to highlight just how huge a problem depression is.

Types of Depressive Disorders

Changing the language around depression is crucial. People who are depressed tend to associate their identities with it by using statements such as "I'm depressed." Thinking of it as a disorder helps dissociate from it. If you had a fever all of a sudden, you wouldn't blame yourself. You'd simply take your medicine and rest and eventually get over it. It sounds hard to think of depression in this manner, but over time, doing so will help you manage your situation better.

Persistent Depressive Disorder: This disorder is also called dysthymia and is present in around one percent of American adults (Koskie, 2018). Women are considered more susceptible, but I've already addressed how data reporting skews numbers. The condition itself refers to low-level depression that lasts for a long time, usually for two or three years.

Bipolar Disorder: This disorder is present in around 3% of Americans, with a whopping 83% of cases considered severe. The disorder manifests as a series of manic episodes where the patient appears to be overly energetic and has a lack of control over their actions. Major depression follows or precedes (or both) the manic episode.

Seasonal Affective Disorder (SAD): As the name suggests, seasonal changes bring about changes in mood. More often than not, the transition from summer to winter causes the condition due to the lack of sunlight. As a result, it is mostly reported in Northern

European countries and places that experience significant swings between summer and winter temperatures.

Postpartum Depression: Despite the huge amount of literature dedicated to pregnancy, it is interesting that not enough has been written about postpartum depression. After all, 80% of new mothers experience this (Koskie, 2018). Hormonal changes and the stress of taking care of a new baby causes it. According to a study, close to 15% of new mothers are likely to experience a depressive episode within three months of childbirth (Koskie, 2018).

Psychotic Depression: Major depressive disorders may be accompanied by hallucinations and paranoia. This is when psychotic depression exists. Patients are usually admitted to a hospital when suffering from this disorder. Rather alarmingly, a study indicates that one in 13 people worldwide is likely to suffer from a psychotic depressive incident before the age of 75 (Koskie, 2018).

Major Depressive Disorder: This is the most commonly reported type of depressive disorder. This condition refers to a single instance of a depressive episode. Understand that sadness and depression are two completely different things. The World Health Organization (WHO) says that 300 million people worldwide suffer from depression, and it is the primary disability that exists currently.

Symptoms

The biggest and most obvious symptom of depression is a feeling of sadness that won't go away after a week or so. In addition to this, patients report a feeling of emptiness for this period of time. Depression is preceded by anxiety, and as a result, the symptoms of anxiety apply here as well.

Constant anxiety accompanied by feelings of restlessness is almost always a precursor to depression. Irritability and an inability to focus on the present are also symptoms. Constantly replaying past events and trying to correct them in some manner indicates depression. Patients at this point will have trouble controlling their tempers and will lash out at those around them. This is just an expression of the frustration they feel about their inability to make changes to situations they find themselves in.

As time goes on and anger dissipates, the patient starts moving away from the activities they used to engage in regularly. As this behavior intensifies, pretty much every thought or feeling that comes into their head is a negative one, and the constant pain becomes unbearable. Thus, the patient tends to disconnect from all emotions and tries to place themselves outside of any feelings. This is a close to impossible task since it isn't possible to be numb all the time.

Sensing the hopelessness of the situation, thoughts of suicide and other homicidal thoughts could follow. As you can see, there are various degrees of depression, and the symptoms vary as the condition gets worse. Physically, all of these mental symptoms manifest as oversleeping, insomnia, tiredness, constant aches and pains, irritability and weight changes, either loss or gain.

Is it possible to nip depression in the bud? The key to doing this is to understand the factors that increase the risk of depression.

Risk Factors

The primary risk factor is of depression genetic. If a person's family history shows cases of depression, they're more likely to suffer from it as well. Childhood traumatic experience such as sexual or physical abuse also increase the risk of becoming depressed. Chronic inflammation or diseases also increase the risk of depression.

Chronic inflammation is an extremely underrated cause of depression. When chronic inflammation has an extremely negative effect on the body, a person is likely to develop a negative state of mind. In younger people, low self-esteem is a major risk factor.

Prescription medication can cause depression

Some medicines inhibit the production of endorphins (the so-called "feel-good hormones") in the body, while others disrupt the digestive system by wiping out the probiotic gut flora. This leads to general irritability, and as a result, the mind-body connection suffers, and depression is the result. Lastly, constant alcohol or drug use only makes depression worse over the long term despite providing short-term relief.

Treatment

Just like with anxiety, the treatment for depression is a combination of medication and therapy. The prescription of medication depends on the severity of the patient's symptoms. More often than not, people who seek treatment for depression end up taking some medication. This is because we tend to take depression seriously only when it gets out of hand.

The World Health Organization states that less than 50% of people worldwide who suffer from depression seek treatment (Koskie, 2018). Studies have shown that relapse is possible after the treatment has been administered. In the case of therapy, relapse is possible for up to two years. Exact numbers aren't available here, thanks to the lack of a strict definition of which state of mind exactly qualifies as being depressed.

As a result, doctors generally conclude that a person who has suffered from a depressive episode once is extremely likely to relapse at some point. A special case is seasonal depression. Given that this condition arises primarily from a lack of natural light, light therapy is often prescribed. Natural spectrum lamps work just as regular light bulbs do, and these often relieve symptoms of SAD.

Consequences

Untreated depression has serious consequences, far more than anxiety and stress. Again, this isn't to minimize the latter conditions but is said more to highlight the seriousness of ignoring depression. For starters, chronic depression almost always results in drug or alcohol abuse of some kind.

Chronic inflammation is also one of the results of untreated depression, and leads to its own consequences, such as contracting autoimmune diseases and other untreatable diseases. While depression is not the cause of these diseases, their roots lie in its existence. Without depression, the odds of a person contracting chronic inflammation are pretty low after all.

Social isolation is almost always present when a person becomes depressed. You will learn more about this, but social disconnection and depression have strong biological links, and the degree of socialization a person is exposed to can directly affect their mental state.

Chapter 12:
Vagus Nerve Stimulation for PTSD

P
ost-traumatic stress disorder is something that can be absolutely debilitating. Understanding PTSD and how it relates to the vagus nerve can help you figure out how best to deal with this trauma. It can help you develop the techniques you need to cope. We will address two exercises that can help with PTSD—using both deep-breathing and cold therapy to trigger the vagus nerve to alleviate the symptoms and side effects common to PTSD.

What is Post-Traumatic Stress Disorder?

Some people are suffering from post-traumatic stress disorder. When this happens, these individuals have repeated, persistent, and terrifying thoughts and flashbacks. They suffering from all of the anxiety of the instance that traumatized them: they may have repeated nightmares. They may find that they cannot focus or work. Even details that are hardly significant to the trauma at all, such as the weather or the sight of something they had seen just before the trauma trigger them, and they have flashbacks after being exposed.

Effectively, these people feel like ethe traumatic instance is reactivated over and over again without their input, and they are unable to do anything other than passively suffer through it. When this happens, they are miserable; it is hard to function when your body is constantly terrified of that traumatic ordeal happening again. You end up living your life trying to avoid things that may trigger the old feelings from resurfacing, but that is no way to live. You should not be living your life in fear of the past.

PTSD and the Vagus Nerve

Stop and consider the vagus nerve's role in response to trauma for a moment. When you are exposed to trauma, such as being attacked by someone or getting in a car accident, your body instantly goes into fight or flight mode. As you know, this is regulated by the vagus nerve, and it triggers the sympathetic nervous system.

This means that the trauma causes a suppression of the parasympathetic nervous system. This leads to an elevated heart rate and the individual being prepared to fight off the threat or run from it. The flight or fight response is considered to be a high activation of the sympathetic nervous system. On the other hand, during lower levels of activation, it is common to see a response known as freeze or faint. When this happens, the individual breathes shallowly and freezes up.

PTSD occurs when there is a lower activation of the sympathetic nervous system for a long period of time. The individual is constantly being exposed to stressors. Through triggering the vagus nerve and reminding the body to get out of fight-flight-freeze mode, you help mitigate the effects of PTSD. By reminding the body to reactivate the parasympathetic nervous system, you shut off all the negative responses. You can lessen the stress by regulating your body's ability to produce hormones to relax.

Diaphragmatic Breathing to Stimulate the Vagus Nerve

When you want to stimulate your nervous system, perhaps the easiest method is through diaphragmatic breathing. This can be done anywhere, and for the most part, can be incredibly discreet. All you need to do is breathe through your diaphragm to trigger the deep belly breaths that you will need if you wish to trigger the vagus nerve's activation.

Your diaphragm is the muscle in your lower belly underneath the lungs that contracts to allow you to draw air in and out of your lungs. People, especially women, tend to fall into the habit of breathing with the use of their chest instead of their diaphragm. Usually, due to vanity or wanting to suck in their stomach areas to appear thinner, this directly alters the way that you breathe.

When can trigger diaphragmatic breathing, however, you will find that you can ease also the sympathetic nervous system response. You can trigger the vagal activity that will help your body regulate itself. Any sort of deep breathing with your diaphragm will work. If you already have the knowledge how to do this, then make it a point to add it in during your day. If you are getting too stressed out, or you notice that your own PTSD symptoms seem to be flaring up, feeling like you are going to have flashbacks or that anxiety gnawing away at you, try to use your deep breathing. If you do not know how to breathe through your diaphragm, try the following:

1. Find somewhere quiet, so you can focus without distractions.

2. Place your right hand onto your stomach, right above your belly button

3. Place your left hand atop your heart.

4. Take in a deep breath and pay special attention to which hand is moving the most. If you notice that your right hand is the one that

moves, you are already breathing with your diaphragm. If your left-hand moves more, you are breathing through your chest.

5. If you are breathing through your chest, take a deep breath, and focus on moving your belly as well. Practice this a few times while paying attention to how it feels.

With diaphragmatic breathing figured out, begin to utilize it in slow breathing exercises. You can use any breathing exercise that works for you, but one that works well is to breathe in and out for five seconds at a time.

You can do this with the following steps:

- Begin by inhaling through your nose slowly. Inhale as you slowly count to 5. If you cannot manage to fit that much oxygen into your body at one time, start with 4 seconds in. Pay attention to how the oxygen fills your lungs, expanding them.

- Hold the breath in your lungs for four seconds.

- Slowly begin to exhale, doing so for the 4 or 5 seconds that you inhaled as well.

- Repeat

Do the exercise for at least three or four minutes at a time. Some people prefer to fit this into their daily routine of meditations or yoga. No matter how you utilize it in your life, it can be useful in pulling the mind out of the fight or flight response.

Laughter to Stimulate the Vagus Nerve

Similarly to the way deep breathing can stimulate the vagus nerve, another commonly used tactic is to utilize deep laughter. When you were inhaling and exhaling, you were able to trigger the vagus nerve thanks to the way the breath moved through your body and your stomach expanded. When you are laughing at something or someone, you are moving your body in a very similar manner. This means that a good laughing session is actually going to trigger your vagus nerve, much like deep breathing did. This means that laughter may literally be the medicine that can best help you.

One of the best ways to trigger long-lasting laughter is finding a comedian that resonates with you. Find someone that you find has a similar sense of humor, and do not hesitate to watch them. In watching them and triggering the response of laughing, you will find that you can activate the vagus nerve, give yourself a workout, and have a good, mood-raising experience all by taking the time to laugh. Keep in mind that this cannot be fake laughing—you need to genuinely laugh those big belly laughs that everyone tries to get out of babies. Your laughing should engage your face, your chest, and your stomach, and the series of movements should be enough to activate the vagus nerve.

Chapter 13:
Vagus Nerve Hacking

T here are some methods of vagus nerve stimulation that you can't do yourself. Instead, you'll need to find a licensed professional. There are also methods of vagus nerve stimulation that aren't quiet exercises but are small lifestyle adjustments that can have big implications for your health. These will be divided into two parts: alternative therapies and lifestyle changes.

Massage Therapy

There are varieties of massage therapies, and just about all of them activate the vagus nerve in one way or another. Massage therapy doesn't just make you feel relaxed but it helps the muscles, bones, and even organs of the body to release pent up tensions. This release of tension brings the body out of the dangerous state and allows the vagus nerve to initiate the healing processes that are impossible when the muscles and joints are tensed for action.

Chronic tension in the muscles can even impact your skeletal structure. Massage therapy has been found to realign the bone structure, which improves blood circulation, nerve function (of all kinds) and even takes the pressure off the spinal cord. Massaging of the feet has been linked to a lowering of heart rate and blood pressure, which in return takes the pressure off the vagus nerve.

Reflexology

Reflexology therapy has its origins in traditional Chinese medicine, but in recent years, it has spread all over the world as its positive benefits are becoming commonly known. The technique behind reflexology is to activate certain pressure points in the feet, which have beneficial results throughout the body. While the vagus nerve itself doesn't extend to the feet, stimulating the pressure points in the feet can do a lot to relax the body and take it out of its dangerous state, allowing the vagus nerve to assume its role as the body's healer in the state of safety. It has also been linked to improved circulation, which does directly stimulate the vagus nerve.

Acupuncture

Like reflexology, acupuncture also comes to us from traditional Chinese medicine. While this healing technique is still being discovered by the West, it's been practiced in almost the exact same way in China and East Asia for thousands of years. Some of the first medical books ever written in any language are books on acupuncture.

This technique stimulates certain pressure points throughout the body, allowing the body to relax and release tension. The Chinese explain this as improving the flow of energy throughout the body. When the energy flow is clogged up, the body falls prey to a number of illnesses. Acupuncture is designed to open up the energy pathways in the body to keep vital energy circulating in a healthy way.

This might sound new age to a Western mind, but from a holistic medical perspective, it actually makes a great deal of sense. In modern medical speak, we think of acupuncture as stimulating certain nerves, with the understanding that those nerves are connected to multiple organs in the body. An acupuncture nerve above the knee or the shoulder, for example, may indeed ignite neural signals that make their way back to the digestive tract, the brain, or the heart, and therefore contribute to whole-body wellness.

Lifestyle and Diet Adjustments

Probiotics

Believe it or not, there are also bacteria that are bad good for you. In fact, there is a whole culture of bacteria that lives in your gut that is not only good but necessary for healthy digestive function. When the health of the gut microbiome is compromised, it can have consequences for the entire body. The gut microbiome is continuously sending signals from the gut to the brain, which is the primary way the brain monitors and regulates healthy digestive function. And guess which nerve carries those signals? You guessed it - the vagus nerve. In fact, a significant portion of the vagus nerve is connected to the gut and its microbiome. If the gut microbiome is compromised, it can shut down the entire nerve.

Probiotics are good bacteria. Consuming probiotics helps to keep our guts (and our vagus nerve) healthy, happy, and fully functional. Probiotics are primarily found in fermented foods. Kefir, kimchi, kombucha, tempeh, miso, sauerkraut, sourdough, natto, and even beer are all examples of fermented foods that are chock full of healthy probiotics that are great for improving and maintaining gut health.

Healthy Fats

There are three ways that the body gains energy from food: carbohydrates, fats, and proteins. These are called macronutrients, and you must consume at least one of the three every day for your cells to survive. While most diets are high in carbs and proteins, the best diet for the vagus nerve (believe it or not) is a high-fat diet. However, a "high fat" diet implies a "low carb" diet. The reason that healthy fats are better than carbs as the body's main energy source is that carbs are pure energy, while fats contain other vitamins, nutrients, and chemicals called ketones, which initiate healing processes at the cellular level. A high fat, low carb diet is the best for a healthy digestive tract and will therefore relieve a great deal of stress from the vagus nerve, which is constantly at work to keep your digestion running smoothly and healthily.

Laughter and Positive Social Interactions

A healthy social life also stimulates the vagus nerve. Laughter is both a physical and psychological stimulator for the vagus nerve, as this is yet another autonomic reflex regulated by the vagus nerve. Positive social interactions do an amazing job in the brain to make the body feel safe, secure and protected. Going long periods of time without positive social interactions can definitely throw the body into a defensive state, which in turn shuts down the vagus nerve.

During positive social engagement, these muscles actual make numerous involuntary movements that signal safety and positive communication to the other person. Sending and receiving these signals, again, stimulates the vagus nerve and causes the body to initiate a number of healing processes. More importantly, these signals cannot be sent or received via remote communication, even through video communication. Therefore, in order to stimulate the vagus nerve, positive social interactions must happen in real life, rather than over the phone or the internet.

Sleep on your Right Side

Sounds weird, but it's actually been found to work. Why? Remember that your heart isn't located in the center of your chest. In fact, it's actually positioned slightly to the left. Sleeping on the left side can be a hassle for the cardiovascular muscles when you sleep, which puts stress on your heart and decreases heart rate variability. Sleeping on the right, on the other hand, gives your heart the maximum amount of space (even more than laying on your back), which improves heart rate variability and subsequently stimulates the vagus nerve and improves vagal tone.

Supplements

Fish Oil

Fish oil supplements contain two chemicals called EPA and DHA. These two chemicals have both been shown to improve heart rate variability, lower the heart rate, and subsequently improve vagal tone. Just one fish oil supplement daily is enough to improve functionality in the heart and stimulation the vagus nerve.

Oxytocin

Oxytocin is another chemical that has been found to stimulate activity in the vagus nerve. Specifically, oxytocin allows the brain to relax and stimulates healthy digestive activity. Oxytocin can be taken as a supplement. Just one supplement daily is enough to stimulate activity in the vagus nerve.

Zinc

Zinc is a very rampant mineral found in a number of different fruits and veggies. Unfortunately, most people don't get nearly enough plants in their diets, and subsequently, don't get enough of this healing mineral. Zinc alone has been found to stimulate the vagus nerve, and it can be taken as a supplement for the optimal improvement of vagus nerve activity. However, eating a plant-based diet that consists of a variety of fruits and vegetables will not only get you enough natural zinc to keep your vagus nerve happy, but it will also flood your body with a number of other vitamins and nutrients that improve gut and organ health.

Serotonin

Serotonin is a chemical that is made in the brain to regulates mood. Serotonin is produced naturally when you are engaged in certain activities that bring you pleasure, including exercises, eating a delicious meal, having sex, or hanging out with friends. However, long periods of anxiety, depression, or drug abuse can cause a serotonin deficiency in the brain, which, in turn, throws the body into a dangerous state and compromises the vagus nerve. If you've experienced severe anxiety, depression, or are recovering from drug addiction, you may want to consider taking serotonin supplements to help the body remain relaxed and in a state of safety until the vagus nerve can do its healing work. Serotonin supplements can be purchased over the counter and have fewer negative side effects than antidepressants or other anxiety medications.

Fiber

Fiber is a nutrient found primarily in plant-based foods. Fiber acts as a gut cleaner, flushing out toxins that have built up in the intestines. When we don't get enough fiber in our diets, certain toxic materials can build up over time and put stress on the gut microbiome, which, in turn, compromises the vagus nerve. A plant-based diet rich in whole fruits and vegetables will naturally get you enough of it to keep your gut (and your vagus nerve) happy and healthy. You can also take fiber as a supplement or even sprinkle it over your food as a powder.

Sun Exposure

Simply getting sun on your skin can stimulate the vagus nerve. Believe it or not, the body is actually designed to absorb a number of vitamins and nutrients (most notably vitamin D) directly from the sun. Some of these vitamins initiate beneficial chemical reactions in the brain and central nervous system. Remember that the vagus nerve is one of the biggest nerves in the central nervous system, so activation of the central nervous system also stimulates the vagus nerve.

Chapter 14:
Vagus Nerve Exercises

E xercise and physical movement challenge you and give you a sense of accomplishment, which directly opposes the miserable feeling that depression causes. In case of anxiety is your issue, exercise gives you an opportunity to vent your frustration at something. Exercise also releases endorphins in your system and helps you feel better. All in all, there is no downside to exercise, and you should aim to make it a part of your daily routine.

Diaphragmatic Breathing

Most people will inhale up to 14 times per minute and in doing so, they have superficial breathing. When you become more self-aware of your breathing rate, you are able to lower the amount to an ideal breathing rate of 6 inhales per minute. This forces your body to practice deeper breathing techniques and fill your lungs to capacity with each breath. It's incredibly easy to practice this routine wherever you may be. I'm practicing it right now as I type!

This type of breathing exercise especially helps to trigger the vagus nerve and turns on its full activation as it is telling the brain that it is now necessary to calm down, even though the nerve itself has not been given that particular instruction directly. In this way, the mechanism is the same as when you close your eyes and tap your eyelids gently. Your brain will perceive each tap as a spark of light shining through.

When we breathe in deeper breaths, we are making use of the lower part of our chests and moving the diaphragm in such a way that it will promote relaxation.

The Power of Stretching

Stretching is used to help naturally stimulate the body and make movement simple. There is a lot you can get out of this. Most people don't realize that they're not only releasing tension within the muscles when they stretch, but they're also focusing their breathing; so it's simple and yet very useful.

A lot of people don't stretch enough, so tension sits there. But a way to naturally start up the parasympathetic nervous system and activate the vagus nerve is to do this: sit down and stretch out your body to promote relaxation and wellness, and from there, stretching will stimulate your entire body.

Try touching your toes, stretching your arms behind your head, pushing them up, holding your arms in the air, or even just moving towards your foot will help with this. There is a lot of benefit to be had. You'll be shocked and amazed, and most of all, you'll be quite happy with the power of this small exercise. You'll feel invigorated and ready for whatever come in the future.

Consider stretching right before you begin your day or at the end of the evening, and see how it helps you feel during the day. You'll feel your vagus nerve stimulated almost immediately.

Weight Training

Weight training might seem weird to stimulate the vagus nerve, but it does work. That's because, when you lift weights, it changes the speed of the body. Plus, through the power of repetition, you get your body to relax. A lot of people thinks that lifting weights is only for big, burly people, but that isn't the case.

Ever just doing a few sets of curls will change the way your body feels. Many people think they need to start with a heavyweight right away, but that isn't the case either.

HIIT Workouts

HIIT, or High-Intensity Interval Training, is a form of workout that require a lot in a minimal period. Sometimes, it involves sprinting; other times, it can be push-ups, sit-ups, or other exercises. The main goal is to do a lot in a short time through spurts.

These spurts cause vagus nerve stimulation. The vagus nerve is usually not stimulated if you're always stressed out. Still, the periods of stress and then relaxation kick the vagus nerve into gear, helping it activate whenever needed.

HIIT workouts are also exceptional because they are straightforward. No matter what you do, you'll feel the difference immediately.

Walking

Walking is an excellent option if you're not going to the gym or don't want to spend time doing HIIT or yoga. Walking is an excellent habit because it stimulates your body and helps with physical fitness and wellness. Your vagus nerve will get stimulated by walking, especially if you live a sedentary lifestyle.

I think walking for 30 minutes a day is ideal, especially if you're unable to do it more. Sometimes, pacing while on breaks is a great way to do it. In any case, walking improves your health and wellness. To help with your physical fitness, walking is a good start, especially if you're not otherwise active.

Jogging is also another good one because that helps with deep breathing. A lot of people, when they start, will get into the habit of breathing in short breaths, but that won't work here. This can make it hard to run, and you might pass out. With jogging, you want to make sure that you're breathing in a slow, deep, and even manner, and focus on this. This will help with your vagus nerve and get you into the habit of breathing deeply. You can also do some running, but it's more high-intensity, and it might be harder to engage in deep breathing.

Jumping

Jumping is another great form of cardio, and your vagus nerve will love it. Jumping jacks, burpees, and other jumping exercises are useful in improving circulation, which can help with blood pressure and your vagal tone.

When you jump, be mindful of your breathing. Try to do it with a deep breath; you'll notice it's a much harder workout, and you'll feel the difference. It increases blood flow, blood pressure, and heart rate as well. Your vagus nerve will thank you for this, and you'll be able to improve your health and wellness.

Yoga

There are not a lot of studies on the effects of yoga on the vagus nerve, but the ones that have been conducted suggest that yoga does increase vagus nerve activity. For instance, a 12-week yoga intervention was found to be more beneficial in terms of mood improvement than walking exercises. A study conducted on the effects of yoga on mood and anxiety found an increase in thalamic GABA levels, which are linked to decreased anxiety and improved mood.

Today, many consider yoga as an effective way to regulate the functioning of the vagus nerve. To practitioners, the goal of yoga in relation to the vagus nerve is to become increasingly flexible. Its main aim is to help people suffering from severe stress and trauma become skilled in switching between the parasympathetic and the sympathetic nervous system with less difficulty. Overall, yoga has been found to be good for improving overall physical and mental health, although more studies need to be conducted on its impact on vagal function.

Aerobics

Aerobics is another higher-intensity exercise, but some variants aren't as extensive or intensive as others. Zumba tends to be on the more intensive side, and there are different classes to try. However, there are other aerobic exercises, such as water aerobics, weight training, cycling, and even some types of yoga.

All of these, when combined, are wonderful for vagus nerve stimulation and great for the body. You'll be amazed at how helpful this can be for the body and how you can improve your vagus nerve. They encourage you to breathe, which promotes deeper breathing and, thereby, vagus nerve stimulation.

Swim It Out!

Swimming is a great aerobic exercise according to most experts, and if you're not a fan of jogging or running, or weight training, swimming is a good alternative. It helps in many ways. For starters, you're submerging your head, which stimulates the mammalian diving reflex, which includes your vagus nerve. It also pushes you to control your breathing as you move. You need to hold your breath but also walk through the water. As such, it is a combination of both techniques which provides correct vagus nerve stimulation. Plus, we all know that swimming improves bodily movement because you're moving about and encouraging blood flow too. You'll notice that as you begin, it's hard to do, but over time, you'll get better. It's a beautiful form of cardio, and it's ideal for properly stimulating the vagus nerve.

Dancing

Dancing is an excellent form of self-expression. Even if you're silly, it can help you feel much better about yourself. Dancing enables you to improve your physical fitness, gets the blood flow moving, and helps you stay active and fun.

There are so many different kinds of dance classes these days. You can do Zumba or other forms like ballroom. Some people even like ballet because it requires muscle control that can stimulate the vagus nerve. They're all fun to do, and they encourage you to move, control your breathing, and let you express yourself.

Even ethnic or interpretive dancing can help. And if it can make you laugh, it will naturally stimulates the vagus nerve in a fun way. All in all, dancing is excellent and lets you feel good about yourself. Consider dancing when you want to express yourself and feel good.

When it comes to stimulating the vagus nerve, these are all practical activities that boost the vagus nerve. Your vagus nerve is vital because it lets you relax the body and helps curb inflammation. But, while these exercises are great for stimulating it, they also get the body moving, which increases the vagal tone. They help offset obesity, diabetes, and other conditions related to weight.

High-Intensity Interval Sprinting

High-intensity interval sprinting stimulates the vagus nerve by waking up the heart and lungs. Doing this one to two times a week will provide the necessary stimulation to the nerve. To do this exercise, run as fast as you possibly can for 30 seconds and then walk for two minutes. This is one cycle. Repeat it for 10 minutes to get a full workout.

Cardio Machines

Treadmills or other walking machines at the gym are great if you don't have a pleasant place to walk outdoors. Especially for those who are living in cold climates, taking advantage of a treadmill at the gym or even investing in one for your home is an excellent way to keep you walking every day, indoors or out.

Jump Rope

Did you ever jump or skip rope as a child? This childhood game is a great way to get your heart beating and your lungs expanding with fresh air. Find a basic child's jump rope and jump for two to five minutes a day to stimulate the vagus nerve. This can be done indoors (of course), but if you can, try to do it outside to get the extra benefits of fresh air and sun exposure.

Resistance Training

Otherwise known as weightlifting, this does more than just grow the muscles in your arms and legs. It also stimulates the cardiovascular system and speeds up metabolism, which, in turn, stimulates the vagus nerve. There are many types of resistance training to explore with your trainer or a savvy friend.

Chapter 15:
Meditation for Vagus Nerve Activation

O ne of the essential ways of activating the vagus nerve is through meditation. Meditation can be used by anyone, even those who do not attend classes. As compared to tai-chi and yoga, which seem to be complex, meditation is a simple approach that involves visualization. The practitioner has to visualize a certain environment that promotes calmness. The main aim of meditation is to calm down the sympathetic action and activate the parasympathetic action of the vagus nerve. If you are capable of sending a signal to the brain that will initiate the actions of the parasympathetic nervous system, you will be in the best position to move on with your life.

To benefit from meditation, you need to choose the right type as but only a few are effective in calming down nerves and boosting vagus nerve action. Some of the meditation techniques used to activate the vagus nerve include:

Mindfulness Meditation: In this type, the aim is to distract the mind from the thoughts that cause anxiety. When you practice mindfulness meditation, the focus is on yourself. You only think about yourself, your body, and your environment. If you want to enjoy the fruits of mindful meditation, you need to observe the rules. First, during mindfulness, a person may discover some frustrating facts about themselves. In mindful meditation, you allow yourself to visualize yourself in a way that you have never done before. One of the most important rules is being non-judgmental. In other words, you are not permitted to judge yourself after observing your thoughts or feelings. You are required to embrace the truth about yourself. This action in itself promotes a calming of nerves.

Some people who suffer from depression only experience nervousness due to the fear of being judged. However, if you can learn to accept your flaws through mindfulness meditation, you will not be shaken by anything. Mindfulness meditation teaches you to stand strong and believe in yourself no matter what the world may say. This is the attitude you need to overcome anxiety and depression. This attitude also promotes the parasympathetic activities of the vagus nerve.

Focused Meditation: Focused meditation is a type where the practitioner focuses their thoughts on a single object. You can choose any object in a room – a chair or a wall. Focused meditation needs intense concentration. When performing focused meditation, you can't release your eyes from the object. Use your mind to describe its different aspects. Think about its design, colors, shape, make, or any other feature. Think about factors that make it special, for example, how it holds weight. This type of meditation is only intended to help you reduce the tension in your mind. After reducing the tension, the body can slowly reduce the sympathetic actions that are leading to anxiety.

Peace, Love, and Kindness Meditation: This is the ideal type of meditation for individuals looking to activate the vagus nerve. The fact that a person may be experiencing anxiety or depression means they need an activity that will lead to the calming down of nerves. There is no better activity than peace, love, and kindness meditation.

You visualize yourself as a center of peace, love, and kindness to the world. In your mind, you visualize a world without violence or hatred where you are the main source of peace, love, and kindness. You visualize yourself extending kindness to people who need it. You stand out as someone who embraces the weak. In your routines, you provide peace and kindness to people who are close to you and try to show them that the world can be a better place. You freely gift people who need help on the streets. You may also visit your enemies and extend a hand of forgiveness. Create a perfect world in your visualization, and just indulge in that peaceful world for a few minutes. When you are done with your meditation, you will be in the right place to let go of all your fears and anxiety. This calming effect activates the vagus nerve, allowing you to live a normal life again.

Simple Step by Step Guide to Meditation

Step1: Prepare the meditation room and tools

For meditation to be successful, you must find a quiet location without interruptions. You can meditate in your bedroom or in an open space. It is important that the meditation location have plenty of fresh air and allows you to enjoy peace during meditation. You will also need a meditation mat or a right-back chair. You may need some meditation music, but it is not compulsory.

Step 2: Position yourself for meditation

Before you start your meditation, ensure you have enough time to complete the session. Switch off your cell phone and only use your watch to set a reminder for timing purposes. Place yourself on the mat in a sitting posture with your legs right in front. Sit in an upright position and allow yourself to freely breathe in the fresh air. If you are using a chair, ensure your back is aligned parallel to the straight back of the chair. This allows your back to be in an upright position, which is perfect for free breathing.

Step 3: Prepare your mind for meditation

You now need to activate your concentration. The easiest way to start concentrating is by focusing on your breathing for about 5 minutes. Do not try controlling how you breathe. Just focus your thoughts and feel how the air goes in and comes out. This will raise your awareness of the environment and allow you to concentrate on the moment.

Step 4: Get into visualization

Once your mind has been prepared for the process, get deep into visualization. You can do this with any type of meditation. You start by preparing your room, positioning yourself, and preparing your mind. Once you are ready, you now focus your mind on whatever it is that the meditation technique requires. For instance, in focused meditation, you may open your eyes and choose to focus on the ceiling in the room. If you know that you'll be doing focused meditation, ensure there is something to focus on in the room. If you are performing peace, love, and kindness meditation, you have to close your eyes and create images in your head. You have to start visualizing your activities as an ambassador for peace to those who need it. It is much simpler if you close your eyes and only focus on the meditation for a given period of time.

Conclusion

Every time we discover something new about the body, we are left wondering at the amazing feats it is capable of, from controlling the immune system to the brain processing information. The body is truly a magnificent system, and each of its parts is an important and fascinating component of that system.

But that does not mean that the body can do everything on its own. We have to make sure we are helping the body function smoothly. Exercising and eating healthy are often repeated topics in healthcare. There is a reason for that repetition. They are important aspects of living and taking care of ourselves.

Certain components of the body require their own special care along with physical exercise and a good diet. For example, the brain needs to feel positive emotions be filled with mental exercises. The same goes for the vagus nerve.

For a long time, the scientific and medical communities never thought to examine the vagus nerve and its complex connections to the nervous system and the rest of the body. When they eventually did uncover its functions, they were surprised at the extent to which the vagus nerve influences the body. As with any new discovery, there was a mad scramble to figure out all the secrets of the vagus nerve and how you should take care of it.

Which eventually brings us to this book. You now have a compendium of knowledge in your hands about the vagus nerve, its influence on the body. Knowing more about the vagus nerve, you are one step closer not only to being aware of its powerful influences but also how you can take care of it.

It is up to you to focus on reducing inflammation in the body, lowering its levels of stress, and using proper routines to improve the conditions of your vagus nerve. It is your responsibility to see that yet another important component of the body is functioning properly.

Our brain alone contains about 100 billion neurons (Shulman, 2019). Yet, as amazing as the brain is, it can't function properly without help from the nervous system.

The vagus nerve isn't the only nerve in the body, but it's undoubtedly the longest. The vagus nerve is the thread that binds all of our inner organs together, facilitating a vast network of connections that run throughout the entire body. Directly or indirectly, everything that happens in the body is connected to the vagus nerve. It's the spark of life that keeps our organs working and our brain functioning. If this nerve can't do its job, then nothing in the body can function the way that it normally should.

As long as the vagus nerve is defensive and tense, it cannot regulate the organs homeostatically. The healing processes happening in a state of safety are disrupted or delayed. The digestive functions are chemically disturbed, and the health of the gut microbiome is compromised.

All the stimulating exercises, techniques, and procedures that facilitate vagus nerve function are designed with one primary goal—

bringing the vagus nerve back into a state of safety. Everyone's brain is different, and not all of these healing techniques will work for you. Some will want to do them every day, while others you may only do them every week or even every month.

You may be someone who enjoys physical or medical interventions, and you may prefer physical exercises and diet changes. You may be prefer psychological interventions and opt for meditations and social engagement. The point is there is a way for everyone.

www.ingramcontent.com/pod-product-compliance
Lightning Source LLC
Chambersburg PA
CBHW050737030426
42336CB00012B/1619